# Setting the Mood with Aromatherapy

## Carly Wall, CA

*Illustrated by Joanna Roy*

Sterling Publishing Co., Inc. New York

*In loving memory of my son Chris,*

*one of those rare spirits who knew how to enjoy life to the fullest*

*and how to share his joy with others.*

---

Edited by Jeanette Green
Designed by Virginia Wells Blaker
Copyedited by Margaret Dietz-Denton

**Library of Congress Cataloging-in-/Publication Data**

Wall, Carly, 1960-
 Setting the mood with aromatherapy / Carly Wall ; illustrated by Joanna Roy.
  p.    cm.
 Includes index.
 ISBN 0-8069-9871-7
  1. Aromatherapy.    I. Roy, Joanna, ill.    II. Title.
 RM666.A68W356 1998
 615'.321—dc21                                              97-51568

1  2  3  4  5  6  7  8  9  10

Published by Sterling Publishing Company, Inc.
387 Park Avenue South, New York, N.Y. 10016
© 1998 by Carly Wall
Distributed in Canada by Sterling Publishing
c/o Canadian Manda Group, One Atlantic Avenue, Suite 105
Toronto, Ontario, Canada M6K 3E7
Distributed in Great Britain and Europe by Cassell PLC
Wellington House, 125 Strand, London WC2R 0BB, England
Distributed in Australia by Capricorn Link (Australia) Pty Ltd.
P.O. Box 6651, Baulkham Hills, Business Centre, NSW 2153, Australia
*Manufactured in the United States of America*
*All rights reserved*

Sterling ISBN 0-8069-9871-7

Preparations of herbs and essential oils in this book are intended to relieve discomfort and distress. Consult a physician if symptoms persist. Carefully follow directions and heed all cautions. Do not ingest essential oils. Author and publisher cannot be responsible for misuse, carelessness, or allergic reactions. Purchase only pure essential oils and herbs without additives and solvents.

# CONTENTS

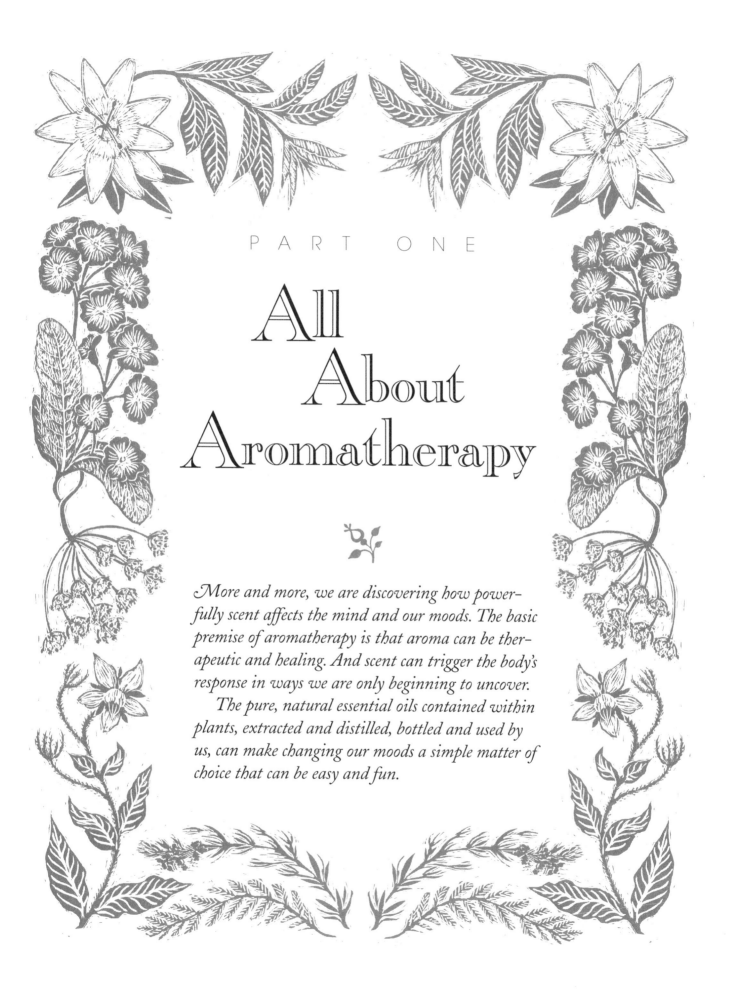

PART ONE

# All About Aromatherapy

More and more, we are discovering how powerfully scent affects the mind and our moods. The basic
premise of aromatherapy is that aroma can be therapeutic and healing. And scent can trigger the body's
response in ways we are only beginning to uncover.

The pure, natural essential oils contained within
plants, extracted and distilled, bottled and used by
us, can make changing our moods a simple matter of
choice that can be easy and fun.

# CHAPTER ONE

# *Mysterious Moods*

*"Be not contented with little;
he who brings
to the springs of life
an empty jar
will return with two full ones."*

—Kahlil Gibran, 1883–1931

Why do we want to "set the mood"? Because we want to experience the best of life, to live it to the fullest and enjoy every second. We don't want to waste our time feeling grumpy, blue, upset, anxious, and angry when we could be enthusiastic, joyful, relaxed, alert, and energetic. We've experienced these happy states of mind, but how can we hold on to them, encourage them to come to us, and banish the bad moods?

We seem to be at the mercy of events and our own swings of feeling. Suppose that a romantic evening would do you and your partner a world of good, but you're too overworked to get out of your stressed mood. Maybe you have a friend who badly needs cheering up. Perhaps someone you know could use a burst of energy and creativity to start a potentially exhilarating new job. Maybe the kids' bad temper and grumpiness have been driving you crazy, and everybody would be better off if they snapped out of it. According to Randy Larsen, professor of psychology at the University of Michigan, most people have bad moods three days out of ten. "Emotional ups and downs are a part of human nature."

## *Master of Our Moods*

Moods aren't tangible. We can't take our emotions into our hands and examine them. We can feel them deep inside, but we can't see them. They are mysterious inhabitants of our minds and hearts. How do we work with something so elusive?

We are all in the same boat, floating on an ocean of feelings and emotions.

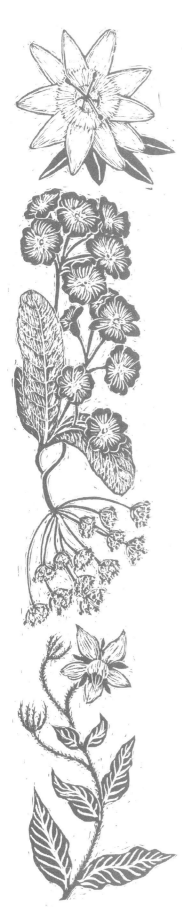

Yet we have the power to guide ourselves, to temper our emotions, and to ride out the storm, if we are willing to learn the methods of aromatherapy. No longer need we toss around rudderless. We can use the healing qualities of the aromatic plants to steer ourselves into calmer waters.

## What Are Moods?

What are moods? Where do they come from? Why are some of us particularly vulnerable to mood swings?

### The Emotional Self

A study done over 30 years ago by Stanley Schachter and Jerome Singer found that first some type of arousal takes place and that this arousal is then interpreted in emotional terms. The emotion "felt"—joy, sorrow, hate, fear, or whatever—creates a state of mind, or mood.

Gerald Epstein, M.D., talks of emotion as a reaction to *stimuli,* emotion literally meaning "movement from." Many factors can act as stimuli to cause emotional reactions.

There are the situations we encounter daily, the outside conditions that force us to react in some way (the grouchy saleslady, the pressing deadline). There are the internal stimuli, the foods or chemicals we take into our bodies. These include the scents we inhale, absorb, or ingest.

"Any outside stressor, from someone cutting ahead of you in the supermarket all the way up to the death of your spouse, can cause a bad mood," says Dianne Tice, professor of psychology at Case Western Reserve University, who has studied and conducted mood surveys. She adds, "It can be so subtle you don't realize it, but waking up in a bad mood can simply mean you are experiencing stress carried over from the day before. People under stress often wake up in bad moods."

She is also quick to point out that mood is affected by weather (rain and harsh weather being downers), financial situations, and the people we meet or know in our lives.

### Men & Women

There are other reasons for changes in mood. Randy Larsen, mood researcher, says, "On a ratio of good to bad moods, there is an intensity difference between men and women, with women experiencing emotions much more intensely but with one exception. Men experience more anger, and much more intensely, than women."

This leads us to theorize that perhaps we are culturally shaped in how we experience emotion. Women are "allowed" to be emotional. Men, on the other hand, have only the avenue of anger by which to vent their feelings and frustrations. How we deal with our emotions seems to be a learned behavior from our parents. If we are taught by example how to handle mood fluctuations, we are likely to have coping skills as adults. If we end up with bad coping skills, even small stresses can overwhelm us and make us bad-tempered and hard people to be around.

## Personality Types, Genes & Hormones

We may also be born with certain predispositions. Researchers believe that people have measurable differences in physiological and emotional makeup. These differences apparently lead to the psychological distinctions of Type A personalities, who are susceptible to anger, and Type B personalities, who are easygoing. Perhaps, too, hormonal changes have something to do with it. Researchers have found that premenstrual and menstrual women experience a marked increase in intensity of emotion. These myriad factors push and pull us in all emotional directions. And what are we to do? We would like to have some control over our feelings without doing away with them altogether. Because we have emotions, we feel, we relate, we react appropriately. Life would be dull without emotional changes. But we would like to make joy and happiness stay with us a little longer, and learn to lighten the burden of grief and depression.

To know how desperate people are to find an answer, look in the telephone book at the list of social workers, psychiatrists, and marriage counselors. Look in the bookstore at the number of self-help books promising success and happiness.

## Stimulants & Depressants

Sometimes we try self-stimulation, with drugs, alcohol, or food. They work for a while. Drugs and alcohol we all know are a dead end. Research has shown that food also can create an addictive cycle. Perhaps we reach for a chocolate bar when battling premenstrual syndrome (PMS), or gulp coffee when stressed. Both these "foods" contain caffeine. Jonathon Scher, M.D., states: "No study has ever linked caffeine to any miscarriages, birth defects, breast diseases, or other health problems. But caffeine is a chemical that does affect the metabolism and mood. The age-old saying of moderation in everything makes good sense in this respect, too."

Elizabeth Somer, in *Food and Mood,* recommends a balanced diet to help level mood swings. Recent research has shown that carbohydrates, both starches and sugars, have a calming effect. They boost the body's level of insulin, which in turn causes the release of a chemical in the brain called serotonin, known for its soothing abilities. But ingestion of too much sugar from simple carbohydrates can lead to many detrimental disorders and has been shown to make mood crashes worse. Food does alter our brains chemically and thus alters our moods. But our use of it has produced too crude and drastic an effect.

### Mind & Body

As Schachter and Singer hypothesized, emotional states all involve physiological arousal. But it seems that there is something more going on. Arousal states seem to cause chemical reactions, just as food triggers a chemical release. One researcher supports the idea that anxiety is associated with production of epinephrine and that norepinephrine release is associated with anger or aggression. This theory is supported by the fact that predatory animals like lions and tigers produce more norepinephrine than nonpredatory species like sheep or cows. And that is the key. What is needed for mood change and control is some type of trigger, a natural trigger that doesn't cause any unwanted side effects.

Even though emotions aren't tangible, we can see the effects of negative or positive feelings on our health. Mind and body are closely connected. In 10th century China, Tan Chiao wrote, "Emotion in the heart is like poison in a substance, like fire latent in reeds." How very true. Clinical studies show that psychological and emotional states influence many bodily processes through the suppression or stimulation of immune cell activity, adrenal gland hormones, and neurotransmitters. Studies at the Ohio State Medical School found that exam stress decreased the function of T cells, which protect the body from disease. We can literally control the health of our bodies by guiding our emotions.

## *Getting the Right Vibes*

### Bach Flower Remedies

Dr. Edward Bach (1886–1936), a British physician ahead of his time, favored a holistic approach to healing. In the 1930s, he felt that standard medical practice was lacking, so he set off on a journey that would take him beyond the bounds of science. He wanted to heal the whole person, not just the illness. "Behind all disease lie our fears, anxieties, greed, likes, and dislikes." He believed that emotions played a crucial role in the health of the physical body. Finally he created what came to be called the *Bach flower remedies:* a method of using a plant or flower's "energies" or "vibrations" to break down the emotional barriers that create physical disease.

9

## Phytochemicals & Essential Oils

While the Bach method uses only the "spiritual" or "vibratory" qualities of the plants, aromatherapy uses their "lifeblood," the phytochemicals (plant chemicals) that physically contain the characteristic properties of the plant: its color, flavor, scent, and resistance to disease. By an extraction process, those phytochemicals are made into the essential oils on which aromatherapy is based. However, herbalists have recently incorporated plant vibrations into their healing methods, believing that they have an effect on a wide spectrum of physical diseases and mental states.

Extraction of the "spirit" of the plant with its physical healing qualities seems to date from early human history. The process was known to the Australian aborigines thousands of years ago, and most shamanistic cultures probably have used such methods. In Chapter 2 we give a method for using the vibratory aspects of plants, and in Chapters 3 through 7 we suggest which of the Bach flower remedies to use for negative moods. I believe that it is an important step toward emotional wholeness to combine two aspects of healing that have been separated in modern times.

## Messages from the Old Brain

"Science tells us that everything is energy . . . In fact, the universe and everything in it is made up of different levels of vibration." So says Dr. John Veltheim, reiki-energy therapist. Science tells us that all matter is in motion. Dr. Richard Broeringmeyer states, "Life is not possible without electromagnetic fields" and adds that if these fields are out of balance for long time periods, optimum health is not possible. Scientific studies have proved that human energy fields are directly affected by activity in the earth's electromagnetic field. Homing pigeons navigate by tuning into the earth's magnetic field through crystalline minerals (magnetic magnetite) located on the surface of their brains.

Humans have similar crystals, located high up behind the nasal passages and near the pituitary and pineal glands. These glands secrete a wide range of vital neurohormones, such as melatonin and serotonin, which stimulate certain areas of the brain, influencing virtually all human functions: mood, sleep-wake cycles, appetite, and sex drive. This limbic area, or "old brain," which controls our emotions, is right in the center of the brain, and the pineal gland is very close to it.

Evidence indicates that the magnetic fluctuations we encounter every day—ROM power lines, computer terminals, microwaves, hair dryers—stress the body and affect mood, as well as cause physical disease. We've heard reports that children living near power lines contract leukemia at abnormally high rates compared with the general population. And is the high rate of breast cancer among female beauticians caused by the continued use of hair dryers held at chest level? The pineal gland is highly sensitive to the slightest fluctuations in the earth's magnetic fields. Why do we have this sensitivity if we don't use it the way homing pigeons and other animals do? We are programmed by nature to receive messages, subtle and yet powerful messages.

## *What Is Aromatherapy?*

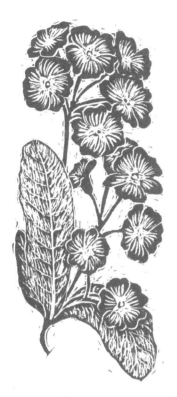

The premise of aromatherapy is similar to that of herbalism: that contained within herbs, plants, spices, and flowers are healing properties. Aromatherapy, however, uses volatile or essential oils extracted from plants in a highly concentrated and pure form, up to 100 times stronger than fresh or dried herb material. It also, of course, emphasizes the power of scent—*aromatherapy* means "healing with scent." Mercedes Hnizdo, clinical aromatherapist, herbalist, and massage therapist, puts it this way: "Aromatherapy is the 'responsible' use of essential oils which rebalances and heals the body, mind, and spirit. It is very effective in changing or enhancing mood states. A whiff of a citrus oil can disperse depression and uplift mood within a matter of moments."

### Healing with Scent

In the 1920s, research into the sense of smell uncovered its enormous influence on the function of the central nervous system. Between 1950 and 1970, Dr. Jean Valnet demonstrated its further benefits in the treatment of mental conditions. Other researchers in the 1970s showed that the essential oils had restorative effects on patients with hysteria or nervous depression. The modern popularity of aromatherapy owes much to Marguerite Maury, the wife of a French homeopathic physician, who developed a set of techniques for extraction and use of the essential oils. She argued that the essential oils act through the olfactory system and through skin absorption to affect the brain. Recent studies have proved that particular aromas do cause brain-wave changes, and since the effects of aromatherapy are measurable, it is becoming accepted by mainstream America. In Europe it has been regarded for some time as among the most therapeutic and rejuvenating of all botanical treatments.

Actually it is a very old story. Scent has always played a part in human existence. Marcel Lavabre, president of the American Aromatherapy Association, asserts in his works that perfumes have been used down through the centuries as medicines. There has rarely been a period when odors have not been important to the care of the body and mind. Anthropologists at the Olfactory Research Fund say that while we in the Western world have become highly visual, it wasn't always so. Other parts of the world still have strong connections to scent. Body odor is so uncommon among Japanese that it once could disqualify a man from military service. The use of fragrant baths to protect and purify the body is common in Brazil. Dr. Margaret Mead, the late anthropologist, found primitive cultures in which tribes actually went to war because they hated each other's odor. In the Middle Ages, alchemists applied barberry-oil poultices to the foreheads of women wishing to conceive, while in 1st century China, madness was "cured" with rose-oil potions. The legend arose in Arabia that when Mohammed rose to Heaven, his sweat fell to earth, smelling of roses, and that thereafter the scent of roses reminded his people of him. It was in Arabia that the art of distilling essential oils was perfected, and much of Arabic cuisine is traditionally flavored with orange or rose water.

## *The Sense of Smell*

Smell is located in the oldest part of the brain (what is called the limbic system) and goes back to a time when living organisms had only the ability to receive chemical signals in order to locate food, detect enemies, and identify mates. As the environment changed, evolutionists say organisms changed and developed, retaining the limbic system as the seat of emotions, sexuality, creativity, and memory. We now possess an olfactory bulb, buried in folds of the frontal cortex and providing a pathway to the hypothalamic and limbic areas of the brain (the old brain, seat of the emotions). High-power microscope probes have revealed a tiny pair of pits, one in each nostril, against the septum an inch inside the nose. These pits are lined with receptor cells that fire messages to the olfactory bulb as scent molecules come in contact with it. It is no wonder, then, that scent has an immediate impact on the emotions. There are six million or more smell receptor cells, with which we can distinguish more than 10,000 odors, and these cells are replaced every 1 to 2 months.

How exactly scent acts on the brain is still unknown. One theory is that the smell receptors respond to the vibrational frequency of the scent molecules. That would be an explanation of why pure essential oils work for healing and synthetic scents don't; lab-created scents can't re-create the vibratory aspects of the plants.

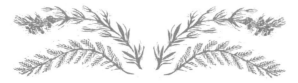

# The Power of Essential Oils

Certain essential oils have been found to have particular physiological effects. A few drops of lavender and neroli can induce calm and a positive attitude by stimulating neurochemical secretions of serotonin. Thyme and tea tree renew cells and protect them by stimulating the production of white blood cells. Geranium and clary sage keep the endocrine system balanced and regulated, lifting the spirit and reducing stress.

Sylla Sheppard-Hanger, with over 20 years of experience in the practice of aromatherapy, relates her observations of how powerful the essential oils are. "Essential oils work best in healing the mind and emotions," she says. "The effect is immediate. Whether we detect the electrical impulses set in motion or not, it still affects the brain and, in turn, causes a change in conscious perception—along with various changes which still occur in the body." Even if we have little or no sense of smell, the effects are still available to us. Anne Hall, a member of the Touch for Health Instructors' Association, reports: "When you introduce molecules of natural essential oils into the air, they coat the cilia in our olfactory system. Gradually, we lose awareness of the scent, but it is still there, and continues to function. This is also true of individuals that have no olfactory perception. There has been research which shows the effects in the bloodstream and electrical systems within the body. The use of carefully chosen pure essential oils not only can be very powerful in the enhancement of a mood or emotion but also has a physiological, biochemical, and psychological effect."

All the aromatherapists I have talked with viewed the future role of aromatherapy as a bright one. Hnizdo states: "In addition to being part of every family's basic health program, I envision aromatherapy being used alongside allopathic medicine at all health centers and hospitals in the United States. This may take time, but it is bound to happen." Dr. Patricia McPartland, certified holistic aromatherapist and hypnotherapist, agrees. "The future of aromatherapy is indeed bright. It will remain popular in shampoos, skin lotions, and cosmetics. Many alternative and complementary healers, including massage therapists, reflexologists, and hypnotherapists, are now using holistic aromatherapy in their practice. I expect this will only increase and we will eventually see aromatherapy being used by physicians." Holistic aromatherapy, she adds, "is a caring, hands-on and natural therapy which uses essential oils and massage for treating a wide range of disorders involving both mind and body. It promotes relaxation, increases energy, reduces effects of stress, and balances mind, body, and soul. It is not a substitute for medical care, though it offers valuable tools for providers working in healing and stress management."

It comes down to this: essential oils can safely and dramatically affect our moods and help us manage our emotional lives. Let's explore how.

# CHAPTER TWO

# Using Aromatherapy

*"What is the worth
of anything
but for the happiness
'twill bring?"*

—Richard Owen Cambridge,
1717–1802

You'll soon discover how many exciting ways of using essential oils and other herbal preparations aromatherapy can offer. Part Two concerns "Dispelling Negative Moods" and Part Three "Enhancing Positive Moods." Along with many choices of essential oils, we provide advice about herbal teas, tonics, tinctures, and Bach flower remedies. These herbal and floral remedies do not use essential oils. All can be very healing when used with care.

Methods of applying aromatherapy are *inhalation* in a diffuser or lamp, on handkerchiefs, or inside sachets or pillows; *absorption* (topically) in lotions, massage oils, hot or cold compresses, perfumes, colognes, or baths; and *ingestion* in herbal teas, tinctures, and tonics. Herbs that are safe for consumption and pesticide-free may be used in all three methods. Essential oils, however, must be restricted to inhalation and absorption methods. They must be used sparingly and cannot be used topically on skin unless well diluted with a carrier oil or with water. Follow all directions carefully. Do not ingest essential oils; drinkable herbal teas, tonics, and tinctures use herbs, not essential oils.

## Important Cautions

Please remember that essential oils are powerful concentrations of plant chemicals and, therefore, very dangerous if mishandled. Never let anyone, especially not children or pets, get into your supplies. Do not ingest essential oils. Never place an essential oil full-strength on the skin (it could burn), and use only the few drops specified. Consult a qualified aromatherapist rather than experiment on your own. Also, heed all cautions that follow (pp. 15–16) as well as those given for particular essential oils found in these chapters. Herbal and floral

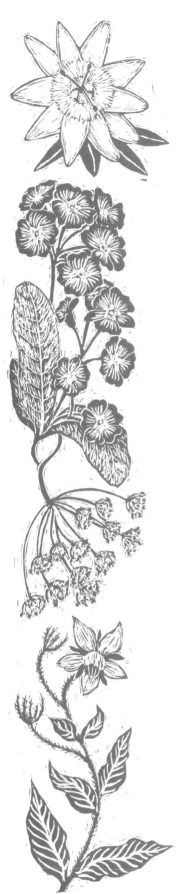

remedies are safer, since plant material is less concentrated, but herbs and flowers' potent healing properties, as well as their interactions and contraindications, must also be respected.

## Just a Drop

We do NOT recommend ingesting essential oils except under the supervision of a competent aromatherapist. (Check the International Federation of Aromatherapists, London, England.) We do, however, give instructions for making teas and tinctures from the herbs (NOT THE ESSENTIAL OILS). An essential oil should NOT be placed full strength on the skin. It could burn you or cause severe irritation. In our instructions for using the absorption method, we specify a few drops in the bath or in a given amount of an innocuous base to make a lotion or massage oil. And inhalation usually requires only a few drops in a diffuser or aroma lamp or on a handkerchief for a limited period of time. *Remember, a drop is only a very small amount.*

> **Note:** 80 to 100 drops = 1 teaspoon = 5 milliliters
> 1 eyedropperful = 20 drops = 1/5 teaspoon = 1 milliliter

### *For Children, Pregnant Women, the Elderly or Sick*

For children under 6 years of age, use only as directed. Always use a half-strength amount for children 6 to 12, the elderly, and the ill. In general, children and pregnant or frail individuals should observe all cautions and be given only the safest essential oils, like lavender, rose, chamomile, and tea tree.

## Patch Test

Before using an untried essential oil, administer a patch test. Place a drop of oil on a cotton ball and brush it lightly across the inside of the person's elbow. If there is no red irritation or itching 15 minutes later, that oil is safe to use.

As for allergies, aromatherapist Elizabeth McNulty advises: "I've never found a client to have an allergic reaction to the true pure essential oils—only the synthetics. For severe allergies or hypersensitivities, I start out with gentle lavender." Stress plays a big role in exacerbating certain allergies, as do suppressed immune function and daily bombardment with synthetic products. The essential oils used for stress relief may in fact alleviate some allergic conditions.

### Overuse

Overuse can cause the opposite effect than the one hoped for. Too much of a relaxant may result in irritation and bad temper. Be sure to follow directions and limit exposure time.

### Quick Results

You get a quick response from the essential oils because, whether inhaled or absorbed, they pass rapidly into the bloodstream. They do not accumulate in the body but are excreted from it in urine, feces, perspiration, and breath. They cannot be addictive and are unlike synthetic chemicals or drugs because they do leave the body so completely. Once you have administered an oil, you can expect to see a change within 15 minutes to 12 hours. The oil will take from 3 to 12 hours to leave the body completely, but its effects may be felt for weeks.

According to Dr. Patricia McPartland: "How fast results can be seen depends upon the individual and situation, whether a severe or long-standing condition is being treated. I have used my lavender blend for allergies and found it relieved symptoms by the next day, the effect lasting for weeks. Clients seem to get relaxed and see a reduction in stress almost immediately. Other more serious or long-term emotional and physical imbalances take more time." Anne Hall adds, "I find that aromatherapy can anchor a positive change in a balanced state for up to 7 to 10 days. In this amount of time my clients seem to have adjusted to the change and integrated it into their life performance."

Barbara K. Bobo agrees: "The olfactory nerves have a short and direct route to the limbic system, so one should expect psychological as well as physiological effects rather rapidly. The surface of the lung has been compared to the surface of a tennis court, and that is a lot of interaction!"

## *Buying Essential Oils*

The extraction of essential oils is a complicated process that requires the right equipment, strict standards, and careful training. It also requires a large amount of material: great quantities of herbs yield only a few drops. While it's possible to make herbal extracts at home that include essential oils, it's easier to purchase what you need. What you will need is a reputable supplier.

Specialty shops and most health-food stores now carry essential oils. Remember, "fragrance oils" are not true essential oils. And beware of the synthetic and adulterated oils commonly used today in the cosmetics and food industries. They simply do not have the therapeutic value of the natural oils.

16

## Purity Test

If you have any doubts, try this test. Place a few drops of the purchased oil on a piece of brown paper. Let it dry (it evaporates very rapidly). You'll know it is pure if the paper shows no spots. If it does leave a stain, go back to where you bought it and complain.

Exceptions to these test results are heavy resinous oils, like myrrh, as well as absolutes and concretes. You want to avoid using essential oils that contain potentially dangerous additives and solvents.

Be cautious if an oil is offered for sale very cheaply. Essential oils ordinarily are rather expensive. Since you use only small amounts, they go a long way. Also, oils exposed to light will deteriorate and weaken. Make sure the oils you buy are sold in dark brown or blue bottles. Keep the lids tightly closed to prevent the essential oils from evaporating. They're very volatile.

## *Using the Whole Plant*

It has many names. In Melanesia, it is called *mana*; in Mexico, *nagual*; in Africa, *ngai*; in China, *chi*; and by some North American Indians, *orenda*. It translates as "spirit-force," a kind of energy that pervades all matter and that many today are turning to as a way of enhancing healing power. It is what Dr. Bach felt as he communed with the flowers in the fields and came up with his flower remedies. Ancient ayurvedic medicine emphasizes holistic practice—treating mind, body, and soul—and speaks of universal energies that can be felt and harnessed. In the first chapter we mentioned the idea that plants as well as everything in the universe vibrate with energy and that that energy can be used to heal.

Indian texts dating back to 2500 B.C. describe how to place herbs on various points on the body so that the energies from the plants stimulate the body and heal those centers. Conversely, experiments done on plants today show that the plants respond positively to being "prayed" over. This corroborates the results being obtained by practitioners of what is called *therapeutic touch*. Refined in the early 1970s by Dolores Kreiger, professor of nursing at New York University, it resembles the early Christian practice of the "laying on of hands" as a mode of healing. It considers the body as a system of electromagnetic energy fields continually in motion, which can be focused and directed outside the body. When any energy path is blocked or unbalanced, the body becomes ill. The energy of another person can be used to heal injury or disease, anxiety, and headaches. And some clinical studies suggest that the method also works on psychosomatic illness as well as lymphatic and circulatory problems.

The whole-plant method is easy to try. Bach believed that by floating flowers in water and exposing them to sunlight, he could release the flowers' patterns of vibration into the water, which transferred the healing vibrations to the person who consumed it. You can do something similar by using fresh plant material for an herbal tea, and after covering the plant material with boiling water, float a fresh blossom or leaf of the tea, and let it set in the sun for several minutes. The plant's vibratory qualities will then be infused into the tea.

### Steps for Preparing Yourself

You may want to try boosting the vibratory energy of whatever essential oil you plan to use, or of your herbal tea. Here's how.

1.  Meditate, or calm yourself. Banish all negative thoughts. You don't want to add negative energies.

2.  Breathe deeply and think about how you want to use the essential oil or tea—for yourself or for a friend or loved one. What mood do you want to create? How do you want to help?

3.  Rub your hands together until you feel heat from the friction. Then hold your hands around the bottle of essential oils or over the teacup. For several minutes visualize a healing energy (in the form of golden light or whatever suits you) infusing the oil or tea. You may also say prayers.

The preparation is now ready to use. The results may surprise you, especially if you compare them with oils or teas that haven't been treated.

## *Using Essential Oils*

*Aromachology*, a term coined by the Olfactory Research Fund, is the study of the effects of odor on a variety of feelings. It combines clinical and psychological factors with the latest measurement technology. Aromachologists agree that scents produce psychologically beneficial results and that those results can be measured. From such findings has arisen the idea of environmental fragrancing—a way of using scent to benefit society as a whole.

### Environmental Fragrancing

Anthony Leardi of Takasago USA said, "We can better modern life by tapping the emotions through the most basic sense, the sense of smell." Alan Hirsch, neurologist, believes that, in the future, odors can be used to reduce error in the work environment and to give employees energy boosts; to raise athletes' morale in the gym; to decrease or increase appetite; and to help in sex, sleep, and a number of other activities. In one study he found that the combined scent of lavender and pumpkin-pie spice caused a 40 percent increase in penile blood flow.

In an experiment at the University of Cincinnati, volunteers performing stressful computer tasks were divided into two groups: one group breathing scented air and the other breathing plain air. Those breathing plain air showed more errors in their work. Mark Peltier, president of AromaSys, a designer and manufacturer of environmental fragrancing technology, installs aroma-diffusing systems in businesses and doctor's offices. For example, lavender may be piped into a doctor's or dentist's office to relax patients. Wintergreen may be used to keep an airline pilot alert. In 85 percent of its projects, AromaSys uses pure natural extracts and essential oils.

## Individual Responses

Environmental fragrancing may have its place, but as Anne Hall says, "Environmental fragrancing to create or change an atmosphere should be an individual choice." We aren't all the same. We are affected differently by different things. To you, the smell of pine may bring warm memories of Christmases past, whereas it may remind me of being lost in the woods some time in distant childhood. The scent of roses makes some people feel romantic, but in others it arouses painful memories of a funeral. So how can we say a certain essential oil acts in a certain way? We really can't. We can make generalizations and then try to pick the right essential oil for a particular person and a particular purpose. Certain essential oils have certain chemicals in common, and these chemicals act upon our systems in the same way, whichever oil we use. Lavender and chamomile both contain cineole and pinene. Both herbs are relaxing and good for relieving headaches. If you don't like one, you can replace it with the other.

## Choosing an Essential Oil

It is difficult to state with confidence that an essential oil does this or that. However, in the chapters that follow, I've chosen essential oils according to what I have found to be their main action: dispelling depression, instilling creativity, or whatever. The list isn't written in stone. You and your acquaintances may have differing reactions. That is why I've listed several essential oils to choose from when you are preparing to "set the mood."

Mercedes Hnizdo states: "We can only make generalizations about the effect of a particular scent based on information provided by literature on aromatherapy and our own personal experience. Still, preferences and dislikes of scent are very individual; and to select the right essential oils, one needs to listen and assess . . . [oneself or others]. The oils must 'fit' the . . . [person], and not the other way around. When it comes to a mood-altering formula, after extensive questioning and assessment, I put him or her through a smell test of preselected essential oils, about 12 to 15. The blend consists of the most favorable three to five aromas. Smell provides a direct link to our 'inner doctor.' The answers lie within, and it is the aromatherapist's task to 'awaken the doctor' within the client. One must listen and observe. The effect of aromatherapy on mood can be almost instant and can be long-lasting as long as the right essential oils are selected in the first place. Also, the needs of the person change over time, and so should the essential oils."

## Blending Essential Oils

You can combine different essential oils to make a synergy (combined effect) of scent to guide your moods, perhaps using one essential oil for depression, one for energy, and one for stress. Don't use more than five different scents in one blend (three is best). Follow the 3, 2, 1 formula: If your recipe calls for a total of 15 drops, use 8 drops of one essential oil, 4 of another, and 3 of a third. This gives you a dominant scent with two undertones, and the scents won't cancel each other out. And don't try to go in too many directions at once. Concentrate on only one or at most two mood states at one time. Elizabeth McNulty says: "I've found that essential oils with similar properties in chemical make-up are the best for blending. It creates a synergy which lets the soul of the plants speak to the human soul." Sylla Sheppard-Hanger points out: "There is the need for what's called individual prescription. In this way, custom blending is effective and more apt to be used and achieve results." Keep experimenting until you come up with a scent you or your client absolutely loves.

### Discovering "Notes"

Dr. Septimus Piesse, a 19th century French perfumer, invented a system of classifying odors according to musical "notes," making up what he called a "harmony of scent." The *top-note* scents have a fresh, light quality and evaporate quickly, so they are the first scents noticed of a blend. The *middle note* emerges a little after the top note, and the *base note* is rich, heavy, and lasting. You can think of them in this way.

- ❧ The top note is uplifting and fresh.
- ❧ The middle note is balancing and flowing.
- ❧ The base note is grounding and nourishing.

Blending an essential oil from each note creates perfect harmony, or synergy.

Essential oils blend well within their own herbal group, whether woody, like pine and sandalwood; herbaceous, like geranium and dill; citrus, like lemon and lime; floral, like rose and violet; resinous, like frankincense; or spicy, like ginger. Also, some groups blend well together: woody with herbaceous or spicy, herbaceous with woody or citrus, citrus with herbaceous or floral, floral with citrus or resinous, resinous with citrus or spicy. Of course, people have their own preferences. A scent cannot be successful unless the person using it likes it. Therefore, first choose several essential oils that might enhance the mood you wish to work on. Then find out which ones you or the person you are helping prefers. If you are making a blend, combine top, middle, and base scents. Narrow your choice to about three alternatives; then follow your intuition.

If you are confused as to what you really need or like, or if the person you are helping is uncertain, you may feel inclined to try one of the following methods of reaching the subconscious mind to make your decision.

## *Tapping Your Subconscious*

Three exciting ways of tapping the hidden recesses of the mind are self-hypnosis, the pendulum test, and applied kinesiology. A great deal has been written about each of these subjects. Here I present simplified versions.

### Self-Hypnosis

Hypnosis induces deep relaxation that puts the subject in touch with his or her unconscious mind. It also opens the person up to suggestion and has been used to control weight and blood pressure, get rid of bad habits like smoking and nail-biting, and treat a number of health problems, including acne, arthritis, asthma, cancer, and ulcers. It has substituted for anesthetics during some surgical procedures. Primitive and shamanistic healers used hypnosis to help heal their patients. Today, many physicians and psychiatrists see it as a dignified science with many benefits.

It isn't hard to learn. It is a common trance state. If you have ever been driving and gotten to your destination only to think, "I don't remember stopping at that stoplight or turning that corner," you have experienced hypnosis. While you were driving, the monotony of the route and the unfolding of the road ahead caused your conscious mind to enter into a light trance. Meanwhile, some other part of you took over the driving. Sometimes television puts us into a trance state (couch potatoes are good hypnotic subjects). Hypnosis has often been likened to the daydream state. If you are good at fantasy and daydreams, you will find it an easy tool. When you want to bypass the conscious mind and talk to your subconscious, follow these steps. Remember, it takes practice. Allow yourself enough time to get good at it before you attempt to use it for your mood program.

### Steps for Self-Hypnosis

**1.** Practice relaxation for several days before going into a trance to ask your questions. Get comfortable. Lie down in a warm room. Take the phone off the hook. You may want to play soothing soft music.

**2.** Tell yourself to relax. Repeat over and over that your eyelids are getting very heavy until they really feel heavy.

**3.** Breathe deeply and close your eyes. Keep taking deep breaths. Imagine you are in a peaceful setting: a soothing beach or restful forest.

**4.** Now imagine that your hand and fingers on one arm feel very (pick one) cool, warm, heavy, or light. Try this on other body parts. When you can do this easily, move on to the next step.

**5.** Now imagine that the peaceful setting has a flight of stairs nearby, which you are going to walk down. Imagine you are getting up and walking down the stairs. Count the steps (to 10).

**6.** When you reach the bottom, imagine that there is a desk and someone is working behind it. See this figure (he or she or it) as your inner self, whether it is presented to you symbolically as human, alien, or animal. Let the scenario play out. Ask about the essential oils and see what information you get. You may also ask other questions. Why am I always depressed in the spring? Why is he or she so hard to work with? How can I have more fun? What type of work do I need to do? You may receive some surprising answers.

## Pendulum Test

The pendulum test is an offshoot of dowsing, an old method. The ancient Egyptians had a tool called a merkhet, which they used in their astrological calculations, in establishing locations for temples, and in survey work. In other cultures, forked limbs from trees were used to discover where metals and other treasures were buried, as well as to find water and even missing persons. Eventually people even held dowsing rods over maps and asked where hidden springs or buried treasure was. Dowsing was eventually relegated to folklore, but rather recently it has been tried again by well-drillers and others.

Pendulums can be purchased in bookstores and crystal shops, but you can also make your own. Simply suspend a key, ring, or some other object (preferably elliptical or oblong) by a thread, string, or necklace-anything in which a lightweight object can be suspended comfortably. The pendulum should balance evenly when held aloft and be heavy enough to produce a good arc when swinging. You want to be able to place your elbow on the table, hold the pendulum up

(4 to 6 inches [10 to 15 cm] from the tabletop), and let it swing freely. Make sure you grasp the string or chain between your thumb and forefinger. Still the pendulum. The idea is that your subconscious mind will move the object—not your conscious self. Practice a few times, asking questions. Remember, you don't move the pendulum. After a few seconds, you may see it seemingly move on its own. The pendulum has three movements: circular, sideways, and up and down. Ask which movement is "yes," which "no," and which "unknown." For each person this will vary.

Now you are ready to ascertain which essential oils are right for you or the person you have in mind. Make a tally by cutting a circle from a piece of paper. Draw lines dividing it up into pie sections with a circle in the middle. Place the essential oils along the edge, each in a different section. You may want to place a lock of hair, a handwriting sample, or the person's name in the middle circle. Ask which essential oil is the most beneficial for this person (or yourself) at this time. The pendulum should be drawn to one or perhaps more oils and will signify this by swinging toward them. You can, of course, obtain definite answers by using the yes and no swings. Ask if you should use a specific oil; if you should use a blend, and whether to use bath, massage, etc. You may even get answers as to what is causing your mood swings.

## Kinesiology

*Kinesiology*, understood here as muscle testing, is being used more and more by aromatherapists to test for the most effective essential oils, to evaluate and balance the body and its energies, and to improve circulation during massage. Sylla Shepard-Hanger says: "I use muscle testing sometimes in my work. It is surprising how accurate it is." Mercedes Hnizdo says: "I sometimes use applied kinesiology as a 'support' method to confirm or verify that the final blend is energetically appropriate or in sync with the client. Any technique or method to help tap into the subconscious mind has my approval, as long as one doesn't tie oneself down to only one method."

And Anne Hall states: "I use kinesiology to identify what is best for my clients, for that moment. Kinesiology is the use of muscle monitoring to communicate with the energy field within the body, the mind, and the emotions. Most of our problems hide in the subconscious on a cellular level that doesn't have a language. The electrical signals in our muscles act as the interpreter. As a 'specialized kinesiologist,' I have training and awareness of healthy physical functions, psychology, and behavior patterns. When a person goes into stress they drop out of these patterns and their energy field is disrupted. Kinesiology shows us how much that energy has shifted to a negative or dormant state and what is being affected. The art of kinesiology can be thought of as a method for tapping into the subconscious mind of the client. If everything that is wrong could be fixed on the conscious level, we could do it with a cup of coffee and conversation with a friend, right?"

A holistic system of natural health care which combines muscle testing with the principles of the Chinese system of energy lines of the body was developed in 1964 by Dr. John Goodheart, a chiropractor from Detroit. According to his scheme, imbalances in the muscles, which are linked to illness, are corrected through the enhanced flow of energy through the 14 pathways, or meridians, of the body. Blockage of these pathways is usually caused by physical or mental stress. Dr. Goodheart's method is a way of contacting that very wise subconscious mind, and some psychologists are using it to uncover and correct emotional problems in their patients. Practitioners believe it is useful in treating headaches, neck and back pain, hypertension, food allergies, and even cancer.

Since it is a complicated system, involving diagnosis of weakness in certain muscles and massage of certain reflex points to direct flows of energy to the weak areas, we will learn merely how to do the muscle testing, which we can use to determine which essential oils the subconscious deems best for us. You will need a partner to do the testing (each can test the other).

### *Muscle Test*

These Muscle Test directions were taken from the book *Allergies and Candida, with the Physicist's Rapid Solution* by Professor Steven Rochlitz.

- ❦ Look straight ahead during tests.
- ❦ Don't hold your breath during testing.
- ❦ Don't strain during testing. If a muscle goes weak, let it.
- ❦ Remove all metal and jewelry from the body, e.g., electric watches, necklaces, and rings.
- ❦ Try to keep the mind blank, with no negative thoughts.
- ❦ Wear loose, comfortable clothing.
- ❦ Take the phone off the hook, and don't test if you are hungry.

The subject stands. The tester faces the subject and places a hand on the subject's shoulder. With the other hand, the tester grasps the subject's wrist lightly and slowly raises it to shoulder level. As a pretest, the tester says, "Tell me your full name." The subject answers as the tester says "Hold" and slowly pushes down, firmly but evenly, while the subject attempts to lock the muscle to prevent the arm from moving toward the floor. Pushing lasts 2 seconds or so. Weakness comes when the arm is unable to resist the pressure. The subject should test strong for correct or true statements, weak for wrong or untrue statements.

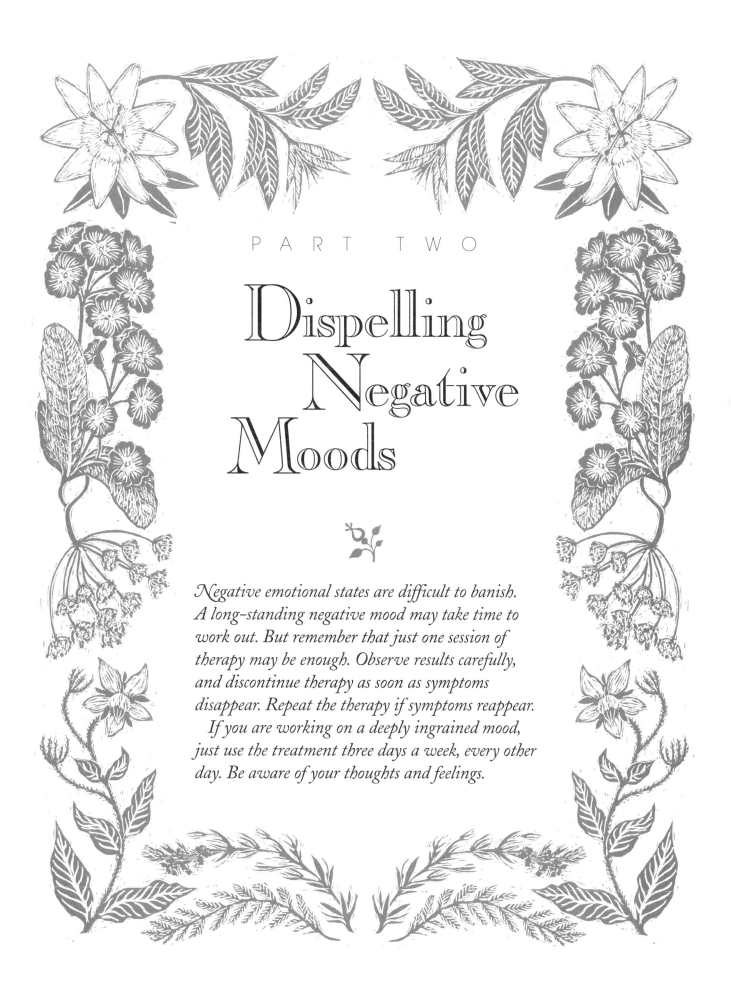

# PART TWO

# Dispelling Negative Moods

*Negative emotional states are difficult to banish. A long-standing negative mood may take time to work out. But remember that just one session of therapy may be enough. Observe results carefully, and discontinue therapy as soon as symptoms disappear. Repeat the therapy if symptoms reappear.*

*If you are working on a deeply ingrained mood, just use the treatment three days a week, every other day. Be aware of your thoughts and feelings.*

# CHAPTER THREE

# Depression

*"We did not dare
to breathe a prayer
or give our anguish scope!
Something was dead
in each of us,
and what was dead
was hope."*

—Oscar Wilde,
"The Ballad of Reading Gaol," 1898

Depression is one of the most common maladies in our society. But we need to distinguish between a blue funk and clinical depression. *Clinical depression* is a serious illness that may require both medication and psychotherapy. Usually people with clinical depression find it hard to function in their jobs and in family life.

Sometimes depression visits us in response to real-life traumas, like the loss of a loved one, a broken friendship, a dwindling business, or being laid off. We go into a period of mourning, as it were, puzzling out the loss or failure. But it is important to our sustained physical and mental health that we revive and be resilient in the face of pain.

Here is a checklist from the (U.S.) National Mental Health Association for symptoms of depression. Consult a physician if you feel five or more symptoms longer than 2 weeks or if symptoms interfere with your daily routine.

### NMHA Checklist for Depression

- A persistent sad, anxious, or "empty" mood
- Too little or too much sleep
- Reduced appetite with weight loss or increased appetite with weight gain
- Loss of interest or pleasure in activities once enjoyed
- Restlessness or irritability
- Persistent physical symptoms that don't respond to treatment (such as headaches, chronic pain, constipation, and digestive disorders)

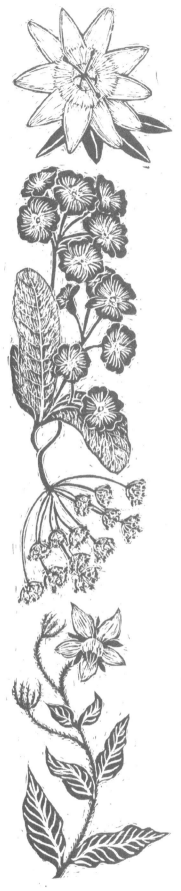

- Difficulty in concentrating, remembering, or making decisions
- Fatigue or loss of energy
- Feelings of guilt, hopelessness, or worthlessness
- Thoughts of death or suicide

## *The Blues & the Blahs*

But what if you are merely feeling "blah"? While the blahs is *not* a serious condition, it *is* very uncomfortable. Almost everyone has experienced the blues or being sad. It's a mild depression. It was once called "melancholy" or "sadness" and in Roman times was thought to be caused by a visit from the god Saturn. One of the main characteristics of depression is a great emptiness, a feeling that there is nothing ahead, no hope. It is accompanied by fear that the awful black, sticky feeling will never leave and that life will never again be active and joyful.

Perhaps we are overwhelmed by a crisis or unsatisfied with the way our lives are going. Tension, stress, and physical illness all contribute. Some allergies and nutrient deficiencies (especially of B-complex vitamins) can cause depression. And there are social as well as environmental factors to consider.

Depression begins with a disturbance in the part of the brain that governs moods. This disturbance causes the neurotransmitters that regulate behavior—dopamine, serotonin, and norepinephrine—to be suppressed. Something happens to keep the brain from functioning normally, probably an overload from a stressed-out life. Normally, if one experiences tension, the brain responds by secreting serotonin. Dopamine and norepinephrine help us to think and act more quickly. That's why a depressed person seems to be "sleepwalking": his brain hasn't been stimulated to secrete the neurochemicals that help us to be more alert. Some people experience *seasonal affective disorder* (SAD); they get depressed in the winter months, when days are dark and short. Research reveals that the bright light of the sun helps trigger secretion of the hormone *melatonin* from the pineal gland. Melatonin helps prevent sadness and regulates our wake-sleep cycles. Aromatherapy works to balance the brain, gently stimulating those neurotransmitters to secrete exactly what we need to put our lives on an even keel.

## Setting the Mood for Elevated Spirits

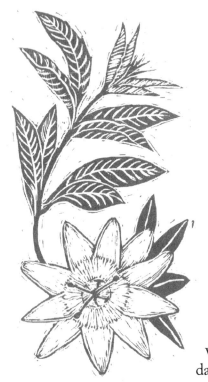

In mild depression, the biggest hurdle is to overcome inertia and make an effort at treatment. That's why I have highlighted the easiest methods of using the essential oils. Most of the oils I've chosen are based on the alcohols, which are low in toxicity, are antiseptic, and can be very diverse in their usage. Many also contain esters, a combination of alcohol and acid. Esters are very soothing and balancing, and it is important to correct the body's imbalance, or what it lacks, when dealing with depression.

As you prepare to set your mood, plan to be alone for a specified period of time. A very light depression may disappear in only an afternoon, but allow yourself at least a week of therapy (treating yourself on alternate days, as we have suggested). This helps the body get back on track and gives you a break from whatever is stressful in your life. Have a notebook and pen on hand, in case you want to write down some thoughts about yourself and your life. If it suits you, gather together a few spiritually uplifting books, or splurge and buy yourself a really fine robe or bed jacket. Hide yourself away from the world for an hour, perhaps in the evening before bed. Make a ritual of it. Try to get a little exercise every day, whether it is walking or something more strenuous. See if you don't feel that the world is a little brighter right away.

## Application

From the essential oils listed in this chapter, choose one that is especially suited to easing your type of depression. Let's say that your symptoms are an awful sadness, headaches, and inability to sleep. You look over the list and decide that lavender (my favorite) has the appropriate properties. It is interesting that many of the oils for depression come from flowers and have a balancing effect. You may want to choose two or three and test your choice through your subconscious, as outlined in chapter 2. Follow the cautions and recommendations for use for the one you choose.

## Inhalation

### Scented Cotton Ball

If you're too down to do much, try the easiest method: inhalation. Carry a small bottle of scent or a scented cotton ball with you. Inhale from it at least three times a day, breathing slowly and deeply for 3 to 5 minutes.

If you see a worsening, or no change, in your depressed state after 2 weeks, seek professional help. Otherwise, be patient and accept that recovery from depression may take time. Massage therapist Theresia Davidson, who uses aromatherapy, says: "Especially those depressions involving past traumatic events . . . require a building up in other ways (such as nutritionally). It is also important to be consistent with applications of the essential oils. And that is difficult for the individual who is depressed. There are also ups and downs to the process, but with care, perceptions can be altered, and although the events cannot be changed, at least the person can gain a perspective from a balanced state." Mercedes Hnizdo agrees and adds: "In my experience, a hyperactive or stressed-out mind with circular thinking and mild to moderate depression is relatively easy to change with the essential oils. It just depends upon the person and severity of the condition. An energetic approach to mood alteration usually works. But here are some tips to choosing the correct essential oil for the situation. For heavy moods, carrying a lot of weight and dragging down the mind, alteration is quicker with the most volatile essential oils or those with 'top notes.' With moods with scattered or overactive thinking, the 'base notes,' which are heavier, often calm and pull the mind down to the center."

Use inhalation with one of the essential oils, and use one of the following methods (absorption or ingestion with herbal teas) in addition.

## Absorption

### Hand Massage

Hand massage is a good way to get the essential oil into your body through the skin, and it also makes you feel pampered. You can do it yourself or apply the hand-massage oil for someone else. It is especially effective on the elderly.

Take 1 tablespoon (15 ml) of either sweet almond oil or olive oil. Add 3 to 5 drops of essential oil (for a blend, add 3 drops of one essential oil for depression, 1 drop of another, and 1 drop of a third). Mix well. Warm the oil in your hands, so that it will be absorbed quickly. Massage well, lightly rubbing the fingers as well as the palm and top of the hand. It is an enjoyable experience and leaves the hands soft and lightly scented.

## Ingestion

### Herbal Teas

**Caution**  Do not use essential oils for teas, use the fresh or dried herb, as specified in the recipe.

**Depression-Easing Tea**  Make a tea from one of these depression-easing herbs, and enjoy it right before bedtime. Use either 1 teaspoon (5 ml) of dried or 3 teaspoons (15 ml) of fresh herbs in 1 cup (240 ml) of boiling water. Steep for 3 to 5 minutes. Strain and add honey or brown sugar to taste.

**Basil** *(also called sweet basil)*  Use the leaves, which have a spicy taste. Basil helps calm nervousness, boosts energy, and restores physical strength. Do not use it if you are pregnant.

**Bee Balm** *(also called Oswego tea)*  Use the leaves and flowers. It tastes much like Chinese tea. It helps depression and regulates appetite.

**Geranium** *(also called rose geranium)*  Use the leaves. Geranium has a floral taste, similar to that of rose. It is balancing and is good for hormone-related depression and PMS (premenstrual syndrome) as well as menopausal symptoms (hot flashes, etc.). It eases tension and anxiety.

**Lavender** *(from* lavare, *"to wash")*  Use the flowers. Lavender has a sweet floral taste. It relieves stress and fights insomnia and headaches (especially migraine).

**Yarrow** *(also called thousand-seal)*  Use the leaves and flowers. Yarrow has a mild astringent taste and helps promote inner strength.

## Bach Flower Remedies

Use 3 to 4 drops under the tongue two to three times per day to treat the symptoms described.

**Agrimony**  For persons who wear a cheerful, carefree mask to conceal deep troubles, rarely imposing their problems on others, and who find arguments distressing, often turning to alcohol, drugs, food, or work to escape pain

**Gentian**  For discouragement, hesitation, self-doubt, depression, pessimism

**Honeysuckle**  Use when dwelling too much on past happiness, lost loved ones, or failed ambitions; no faith in the future

**Mustard**  Helpful for gloom or despair, a "dark cloud" that comes and goes for no known reason

**Sweet Chestnut**  For people feeling at the end of endurance, in great mental despair and seemingly unbearable anguish

# Elevating Essential Oils

## Allspice  (Pimenta dioica)

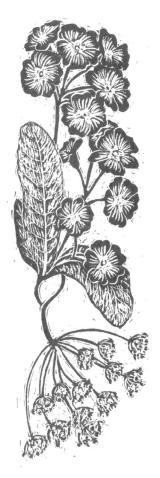

**Application**  Inhalation; small amounts in massage
**Note**  Base, grounding, spicy
**Caution**  Allspice can cause skin irritation. Use low concentrations in massage oils.
**Background**  In the 14th and 15th centuries, the search for unusual spices sent travelers to the West Indies, where they discovered a little tree whose taste and aroma were an exotic blend of cinnamon, clove, nutmeg, and pepper. Soon it was dubbed "allspice." The unripened berries contain the greatest amount of essential oil.

The English naturalist John Ray called it "sweet-scented Jamaica pepper." An evergreen tree that grows in the West Indies and South America, it is cultivated in Jamaica and Cuba. Used to flavor foods and alcoholic drinks as well as soft drinks, it is also popular in perfumes and soaps for its spicy and oriental scent.
**Use**  Allspice is used for depression, nervous exhaustion, neuralgia (sharp pain along the course of a nerve), tension, and stress. Perhaps that's why it has come to symbolize compassion. It is said to be an instant pick-me-up.
**Blend** with spicy scents, like patchouli and neroli, and with ylang-ylang, lavender, ginger, and geranium.

## Ambrette  (Abelmoschus moschatus)

**Application**  Any
**Note**  Base, grounding, floral
**Background**  Ambrette, native to India and now cultivated widely, is an evergreen shrub with kidney-shaped seeds that yield a musky, sweet, flowery scent. The seeds are used in Eastern countries as a domestic spice, in China as a headache remedy, and in perfumes as a musk substitute. The oil can be very expensive.
**Use**  Good for depression accompanied by tension and stress. Considered a nervine, it eases anxiety and promotes a warm, sensuous feeling.
**Blend** with jasmine, lemon, geranium, and any oriental scent.

## *B a s i l*   *(Ocimum basilicum)*

( also called SWEET BASIL)

**Application** Inhalation

**Note** Top, uplifting, herbaceous

**Caution** Pregnant women should not use basil. It can be toxic, so prolonged use is not recommended. Do not use more than 3 drops of essential oil per day.

**Background** Basil was regarded very suspiciously when it first came to Europe, probably because overuse can cause headaches instead of banishing them. However, it is still considered one of the best nerve tonics available. It originated in Asia and is now cultivated throughout the world. In ancient Greece it was considered the herb of kings. It has been used extensively in ayurvedic medicine.

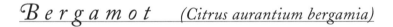

**Use** John Gerard, the 16th century herbalist, wrote, "The smell of basil . . . taketh away sorrowfulness," and he is right. It has long been used to treat melancholy. It is soothing and balancing, yet uplifting, and it chases away sadness. It promotes happiness and stimulates and clears the mind. Helpful for concentration, it banishes mental fatigue, boosts energy, and restores strength both mentally and physically. It banishes headaches. It is antiseptic and warming, but has a cool quality. It helps restore the adrenal glands after extreme stress.

**Blend** with hyssop or bergamot.

## *B e r g a m o t*   *(Citrus aurantium bergamia)*

**Application** Inhalation

**Note** Top, uplifting, citrus

**Caution** Bergamot can cause sun sensitivity. Avoid sun and the tanning salon after using it. Don't use more than 3 to 6 drops daily for skin preparations. Do not take it over long periods of time. Do not ingest this essential oil.

**Background** Bergamot has been used widely in the perfume and cosmetic industries and is a principal ingredient in the classic eau-de-cologne. It also flavors the famous Earl Grey tea. Named after the Italian city where it was first sold, it has been used in Italian folk medicine for years. The small fruits resemble oranges and have a citruslike fragrance at once fruity and sweet. Don't confuse this essential oil with the North American herb bee balm (also sometimes called bergamot).

**Use** Bergamot is uplifting, like the other citrus scents, but has a warm, soft quality. It is a good essential oil for convalescents, since it builds strength both emotionally and physically. It is good for either dry or oily skin. It regulates appetite, helps frazzled nerves, improves mental clarity, and helps relieve anxiety. It is calming and balancing and has analgesic qualities. It is a sedative and therefore good for insomnia.

**Blend** with chamomile, lavender, cypress, and all other citrus oils.

## Cananga  (Cananga odorata macrophylla)

**Application** Any

**Caution** Those with very sensitive skin may experience a reaction to the sun.

**Note** Middle, balancing, floral

**Background** A tall tropical tree that flowers all year, the cananga is very similar to the ylang-ylang and bears similar large, fragrant flowers. However, it grows in different areas from the ylang-ylang and has a slightly different property. It is native to the Far East: Java, Sumatra, and Madagascar. The rather heavy essential oil is a balancing scent useful for depression.

**Use** Cananga oil is good for anxiety-ridden depression and other stress-related complaints, and it helps restore sexual feelings. A great sedating tonic, it helps dispel hysteria.

**Blend** with warm oriental scents.

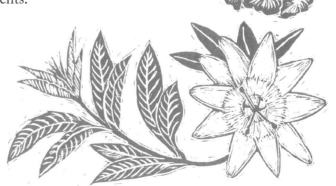

# *Geranium*   (*Pelargonium graveolens*)

**Application**  Any; good in skin lotions
**Note**  Middle, balancing, floral
**Background**  Its delicate roselike scent, somewhat
rich and minty, is one of the most popular in
aromatherapy, and it is often combined with
the costly true rose oil. Many beauty and
cosmetics products contain it, and it is a
traditional flavor in food and drink. A cheerful little plant with fuzzy green leaves, it is a
perennial in warmer climates but must be
brought indoors in colder areas. It can grow up to
1½ feet (0.5 m). Grandmothers of yore saved the
leaves to flavor cakes and sugars for special occasions.
The essential oil is produced in Egypt, Russia,
and China.

**Use**  Rose geranium soothes and calms the most world-weary persons. Relaxing,
balancing, and an uplifting antidepressant, it is good for those experiencing
emotional extremes. It aids in the hormone-related problems of menopause
(eases hot flashes). It also has the ability to enhance sensual feelings. A skin
rejuvenator, it is good for all skin problems—acne, eczema, shingles, wounds,
facial neuralgia—because of its antiseptic and antiinflammatory qualities.
**Blend** well with citrus oils, lavender, or jasmine.

# *True Lavender*   (*Lavandula angustifolia*)

**Application**  Any
**Note**  Middle, balancing, floral
**Background**  The clean, fresh scent of this plant yields perhaps the most versatile of the essential oils. Aptly, its Latin name *lavare* means "to wash," and it
washes away not only physical but mental impurities. For centuries it has been
used for bathing as well as for washing and scenting linens. The Romans used
it to scent the water in their public baths. The Greeks claimed that the scent
of lavender could calm lions and tigers. Lavender water is the oldest of
English perfumes.
**Use**  Use the flower buds in tea for headaches and nervous exhaustion. The
essential oil is soothing, balancing, uplifting, and good for depression and irritation. Lavender is a relaxant that brings peaceful feelings and dispels melancholy. It enhances clear thinking. Good for relieving stress, shock, heart palpi-

tations, dizziness, and negative thinking, it also calms PMS-related symptoms. The safe, gentle oil is very healing to the skin and good in massage oils and bath water.

**Blend** with citrus, rose, and most oils.

# Sandalwood *(Santalum album)*

**Application** Inhalation, absorption

**Note** Base, grounding, woody

**Caution** Do NOT ingest the essential oil, since it can be a kidney irritant. Do not use it for longer than 4 weeks at a time.

**Background** Sandalwood is highly prized in the manufacture of incense and perfumes. The slow-growing tree is found in India, southern China, and the Pacific Islands. Sandalwood is combined with rose in the classic Indian attar. The Egyptians used it in their embalming ceremonies. It was a popular building material for temples throughout its growing region because the wood exuded a rich and powerful, yet soft and mellow, woodsy, warm scent to worshippers who stepped inside. It is favored in meditation for the harmonious calm it bestows. It was used for thousands of years as a cooling remedy and is mentioned in the epic poems of India.

**Use** Sandalwood is a good scent for men, especially those with Type A personality (tense and edgy). It balances the emotions, calms and energizes, and brings harmony while promoting acceptance and openness. It is an antidepressant, an antiseptic, and a sedative tonic that lulls the conscious mind. It heightens mental clarity, concentration, and sexual interest. It is good also for women with postnatal depression. The Japanese call it *sendan,* "bringer of joy." It gives people who want to isolate themselves the desire to be with people again. Be sure to get the true essential oil that comes from the Mysore province of India, since others are often adulterated.

**Blend** with rose, lavender, and jasmine.

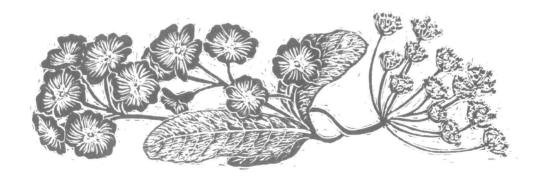

# *Yarrow*  *(Achillea millefolium)*

**Application** Any

**Note** Top, uplifting, herbaceous

**Caution** Avoid yarrow during pregnancy. In rare cases it causes skin reactions. If used for a prolonged period, it can cause sun sensitivity.

**Background** It symbolizes health. In ancient China it was a sacred herb, and the stalks are traditionally used in the *I Ching* to help in divination. The ancient Saxons made amulets containing it, and it has often been associated with witches, from which comes its name "devil's nettle." The Shakers, however, used the feathery green herb for more down-to-earth business as a stimulant and tonic. It is an antiallergenic containing azulene, an antiinflammatory. The oil has a fresh, green, camphorlike odor and is steam-distilled from the dried leaves.

**Use** Premenstrual discomfort affects up to 95 percent of women to some degree, says the National Women's Health Resource Center. With it come the psychological symptoms of depression and mood swings. Yarrow can help relieve PMS, with accompanying depression and mood swings, as well as menstrual irregularity and menopausal symptoms. For depression resulting from inability to make decisions during a major life upset, such as during mid-life crisis, career change, or divorce, yarrow is the herb of choice. It is balancing and is good for stress, headaches, and hypertension. Yarrow has the ability to promote inner as well as physical strength. It is also a great skin healer.

**Blend** with St.-John's-wort, ylang-ylang. Yarrow blends well with St.-John's-wort *(Hypericum perforatum),* which is reportedly good in easing depression accompanied by expressed or unexpressed anger.

**Massage Oil** take a small handful of St.-John's-wort leaves and add it to 1 cup (240 ml) of peanut oil (make sure the leaves are covered). Cap it tightly, and set it in a sunny window for 2 weeks. Strain. To 1 fluid ounce (30 ml) of this oil add 5 to 8 drops of yarrow essential oil. Add a few drops of vitamin E, and shake to blend. This makes a good hand lotion and all-over body massage oil.

# CHAPTER FOUR

# Grief & Sadness

*"Can I see another's woe,
and not be in sorrow too?
Can I see another's grief,
and not seek
for kind relief?"*

—William Blake, *Songs of Innocence*
"On Another's Sorrow," 1789

Survival is the task of the grieving. What is needed is the courage to keep on keeping on, to do what has to be done to continue with our lives. The death of a spouse, child, parent, friend, or even pet; a long illness or pronouncement of illness; a divorce or any major separation; these are deep losses that result in our having to pick up the pieces and start all over again. It is hard work.

Elizabeth Kübler-Ross in *Death: The Final Stage of Growth* (1975) stated, "Facing death means facing the ultimate question of the meaning of life." This is true for the one dying and for the one left behind. It is heavy stuff, and it takes time to sort it all out and to deal with the emotional trauma it brings.

## Loss & Grieving

Our understanding of the grieving process is slowly evolving. In 1942, six weeks was considered a normal period of mourning. Studies in the 1960s lengthened the expected grieving period to 6 months. In the 1970s it was lengthened to a year. Some psychologists now propose that we allow a full 2 to 3 years for complete grief resolution. Kübler-Ross was a pioneer in the study of the behavior of the dying and grieving. She has devoted most of her life to helping those facing death and has observed that they experience a series of reactions that she has described as "the five stages of grief." These stages are a natural process that must be gone through to come to terms with death and grief. Colin Murray Parkes, author of *Bereavement: A Study of Grief in Adult Life*, borrowed and built on Kübler-Ross's five-stage guide and uses it to assess the stages of grieving.

But this guide is only that, a guide. Like everything else, grieving is done individually, at one's own speed, in one's own way. We never forget a great loss, but it does force us to grow and change. Eventually we learn to pick up the pieces and go on, taking with us the lessons we have learned: perhaps a more mature view of life and what it really means.

It is important to note, too, that the phases of grief seldom follow each other in regular order. One day, you will be angry and depressed, another day, weepy or in denial. The time frame can be minutes or hours or day to day. This is natural. The guide lets you know that what you are going through is part of a process, and it gives you a timetable to refer to. Grief and sadness can become abnormal, if you hang onto them for too long. You know this has happened when your day-to-day life becomes dysfunctional. When you have worked through our sadness, tears, depression, emptiness, and despair, normally you don't forget, but you let go. But sometimes sorrow and pain are a tie to a lost loved one, a way of continuing to possess a person or situation. Then is the time to seek help. In releasing what you have lost, you face the world honestly, and that is best for you and for the others in your life.

Aromatherapy cannot take away the grief, but it can help make the passage through all the transitional stages more comfortable. If counseling is needed, aromatherapy can supplement it. It is also important to eat right and exercise regularly. Psychotherapists recommend not making any major decisions—a job change, a move to a new place—within the first year. The first year is a wave of emotional ups and downs.

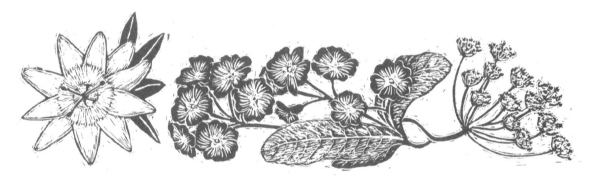

## Stages of Grief

Here is a model of Parkes's stages of grief, modified to include the essential oils specifically suited to the symptoms of each stage. Judge which stage you are going through at a particular moment and which essential oils are best for you at that time. As your moods and feelings change, so will your choice of an essential oil.

**First Stage, Alarm or Shock**  The first reaction to sudden or unexpected news, or even expected news, of a death is alarm or shock. The finality of death, of loss, and of your own mortality, as well, are brought home to you. You may react with tears, wailing, or even stoic silence. You should expect sleep disturbances—either experiencing too much or too little sleep and feeling weariness and numbness. During this period, which lasts about 2 weeks, you will feel as though you are "falling apart."

*Recommended Essential Oils*  Choose an essential oil that aids in reducing hysteria, insomnia, or exhaustion.

**Second Stage, Searching**  You long for the person you have loved and lost and momentarily forget your loss. You may hear a joke or hear about a special event and want to tell your loved one about it, but suddenly you remember that he or she is gone. If divorced, you find yourself driving "home," then remembering that you now live in another place. You miss or yearn for old habits and routines. This stage may last from 4 to 6 weeks or even up to a year.

*Recommended Essential Oils*  Choose essential oils that help balance moods, improve memory, or clear the mind.

**Third Stage, Mitigation**  As the searching phase comes to an end, the sharp pain lessens, but depression and deep despair set in. The loved one is gone, resigned to memory. Grieving dreams become vivid. To get in touch with your feelings, you might keep a dream journal, even write letters to the person you have lost. It may help to go to the graveside and have imagined conversations with the dead person.

*Recommended Essential Oils*  Choose essential oils that are good for depression (chapter 3) or grief (this chapter). You might try helichrysum or clary sage to enhance dreams, and use the oils in chapter 10 to encourage restful sleep.

**Fourth Stage, Anger & Guilt**  After 5 or 6 months, you enter the stage of emotional turmoil. You question, What if I had done this or that? What if this or that had happened? It is a time of guilt about things said or not said, done or not done. It is also a time of anger at oneself, God, the deceased or the one who left, the hospitals and doctors, and the world in general. You feel both guilt and anger at going on alone. During this period you must talk with others about your feelings; you need good friends who listen.

*Recommended Essential Oils*  Choose essential oils that clarify your thinking. Blend any oils in chapter 10 (for anger) with the oils in this chapter.

**Fifth Stage, Identity & Recovery**  Sometimes within a year, sometimes after two or three years, new patterns of life start to form. You take a tentative step forward, then, as often as not, two steps back. Sometimes you forge ahead, then falter and retreat for a while. You may anticipate going out to dinner, then feel overwhelmed when the time comes.

*Recommended Essential Oils* Choose strengthening and balancing essential oils, as well as those that encourage hope and a belief in a brighter future.

## Setting the Mood for Comforting Sadness & Grief

Choose one of the following methods to use daily: absorption and inhalation through a soothing bath, Bach flower remedies, or hot forehead compresses.

### Absorption & Inhalation

*Soothing Baths*

A relaxing and soothing bath enables you to inhale essential oils while absorbing them through the skin. Choose one or a blend of those below. Add the specified number of drops, never exceeding 6 to 12 drops (total per bath), to 2 tablespoons (30 ml) of cold-pressed vegetable oil (for a moisturizing bath) or 2 tablespoons (30 ml) of baking soda (for a skin-soothing bath).

**Caution** Do not exceed the maximum of 6 to 12 drops of essential oil (total) in a full tub of bathwater. Use still less of the powerful or sedating essential oils (2 or 3 drops total) for a full tub of bathwater. Be careful not to use more than the recommended amount of any essential oil.

**Damask Rose** 2 to 3 drops (powerful; do not use more)

**Hyssop** 5 to 10 drops

**Marjoram** 6 drops only (very sedating; avoid if you have low blood pressure)

**Orange Blossom** 6 to 12 drops

**Petitgrain** 6 to 12 drops

**Scotch Pine** 2 to 3 drops (powerful; do not use more)

Have warm, fluffy towels nearby, as well as uplifting and calming music. You may want to take your bath about an hour before bedtime. If you like, use candles with the same scent as your bath. Bathe in dimmed light, for you are emotionally overloaded and need to turn off the world, if only for 20 minutes. To help another person who has recently experienced a loss, you might make up a gift basket filled with premixed essential oils, towels, a cassette tape, and candles, along with instructions.

Your water should be warm to hot. Add the 2 tablespoons (30 ml) of mixture to the running water, and swish it around. Soak yourself for about 20 minutes. During this time, be conscious of your breathing. Take deep, slow breaths, holding each breath for 2 seconds, then slowly exhaling. Concentrate on calming and centering yourself.

### Bach Flower Remedies in the Bath

If you want to use the Bach flower essences, you can add 20 drops directly to the bath. Since these are not aromatic, you may, if you wish, use them along with the essential oils. Here are the five I would recommend. Choose the one that seems best suited to your situation.

**Chicory** overinvolvement in others' lives, wanting loved ones nearby constantly, possessiveness

**Gorse** hopelessness, despair

**Honeysuckle** too great dwelling on the past, lost loved ones, or unrealized ambitions

**Olive** mental and physical exhaustion from burdensome or adverse conditions, illness, or ordeal

**Star of Bethlehem** trauma of bad news, loss of a loved one, fright, or accident; inconsolability, grief

### Hot Forehead Compresses

A compress is good to use on days when you don't want to take a scented bath or when you feel too overwhelmed to make the effort. Put hot (not scalding) water into a bowl. Choose your essential oil. Good choices from this chapter are celery seed, coriander, helichrysum, myrtle, and Scotch Pine. Add 6 drops to the water, and swirl them around to mix. Place a thick dish towel in the water, wring it out, and apply it to your forehead. Keep your eyes closed and the cloth in place for 15 to 20 minutes. You can do this several times a day, if necessary.

### Scented Lightbulb

Or put several drops of the essential oil on an unlit lightbulb, then turn on the light. The heat from the bulb will soon make the scent fill the room. Close your eyes and relax, inhaling the scent for 15 to 20 minutes.

## Ingestion

### Tinctures & Herbal Teas

**Grief-Easing Tinctures** Sometimes, an herbal tincture is the easiest and best way to get comfort fast. Use ½ eyedropperful (10 drops, or 0.5 ml) under the tongue as needed. To make a grief-easing tincture, choose one or more of the herbs below. Add 1 cup (240 ml) of fresh herbs, or ½ cup (120 ml) of dried, to 2 cups (480 ml) of vodka or brandy. For a multiherb tincture use equal amounts of each herb. Place the tightly closed jar of tincture in a sunny window for 2 weeks. Strain and store.

### Feverfew   (Chrysanthemum parthenium)

Feverfew shares some properties with aspirin and traditionally is used to treat migraines. It is bitter but warming, is a relaxant, and induces sweating. It is good for melancholy. Use the flowers and leaves and mix with a more pleasant herb, like peppermint or lavender.

**Caution**  Do not take this with blood-thinning drugs since it affects blood clotting rates.

### Hyssop   (Hyssopus officinalis)

Hyssop clears the head and strengthens the thought processes. A warming nervine, it is uplifting, good for hysteria, calming to feelings of guilt, and gently relaxing.

**Tea**  Hyssop also makes a good tea that helps balance blood pressure. Add 1 teaspoon (5 ml) of dried tops and/ or flowers to 1 cup (240 ml) of boiling water. Let this steep for 5 to 10 minutes. Strain. Drink no more than 3 cups (720 ml) per day.

**Caution**  Overdosing can cause convulsions, especially in epileptics. Do not give hyssop to pregnant women.

### Passionflower   (Passiflora incarnata)

This is a tranquilizing yet invigorating herb that restores balance and improves concentration. Michael Weiner writes that it "may be our best tranquilizer." It is quite effective for states of nervous agitation, and it regulates mood and sleep, producing deep sleep without a hangover the next day. It works well for over-weight, harried, or weakened individuals and is good for chronic pain. Children over 2 years or weakened individuals can be given 5 drops (0.25 ml) up to twice a day in times of high stress, especially if the tincture is made with the addition of chamomile.

It is important to know that the tonic flavornoids are extracted in alchohol only. The leaves are used. It combines well with valerian root.

**Caution**  Do not give this to children under 2 years old. Pregnant women should take low doses only.

### Skullcap   (Scutellaria laterifolia)

Skullcap is quite good for nervous disorders, insomnia, unrest, depression, nightmares, agitation, and restless sleep. It renews while relaxing, and its sooth-ing influence lasts a long time. The whole plant is used. Overdosing or prolonged use can cause headaches, stupor, or a feeling of heaviness. It combines well with valerian and passionflower.

### Vervain (Verbena officinalis)

Vervain is one of the druids' most sacred herbs and was used to purify the homes and temples of the Romans. It is also one of Dr. Bach's original twelve flower remedies for mental stress and insomnia. It is a relaxant, a sedative, and a nervine. It promotes sweating and is used for nervous exhaustion and depression. It is gathered when it flowers in the summer.

**Caution** Avoid vervain in pregnancy.

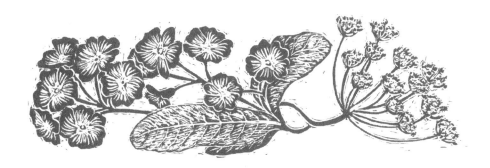

# Softening Sadness & Grief with Essential Oils

## Celery Seed (Apium graveolens)

**Application** Massage, hot compresses, herbal extract

**Note** Base, grounding, spicy

**Caution** Since celery seed can cause sun sensitivity, don't apply it immediately before going out in the sun. Avoid it in pregnancy.

**Background** A cooling and sedating essential oil, celery seed is produced mainly in India, the Netherlands, China, Hungary, and the United States. It is grown worldwide as a garnish and a seasoning for soups and stews. Celery seed is also an ingredient in cosmetics and perfumes. It has a spicy, warm, sweet, long-lasting odor. Its diuretic qualities help rid the body of toxins, and it acts as an antioxidant.

**Use** Because it eliminates toxins, it is good for people who have been neglecting themselves. While it quiets the nervous system, it stimulates the metabolism and increases awareness. It relieves stress-related fatigue, and the essential oil is sedating.

**Blend** with pine, lavender, and coriander.

## Coriander  *(Coriandrum sativum)*

### (Also called CHINESE PARSLEY)

**Application**  Any, especially inhalation

**Note**  Top, uplifting, spicy

**Caution**  Large doses can cause stupor.

**Background**  Coriander seeds have been found in ancient Egyptian tombs. The seeds and leaves of the strongly aromatic annual herb are used widely today as a garnish and spice, especially in Central Europe and Russia. It has a sweet, musky, yet spicy scent and is cultivated throughout the world. It is used as a flavoring in digestive remedies and medicinals. During World War II the seeds were made into what was called sugar drops by being coated with pink or white sugar. These sugar drops were thrown from carnival wagons into crowds. Later, this practice was regarded as wasteful, so bits of colored-paper confetti replaced the candies.

**Use**  A warming essential oil, coriander restores energy and appetite, relieves headaches, and helps restore memory. It also helps to instill courage and give one the feeling that life can be handled one step at a time.

**Blend**  with clary sage, bergamot, sandalwood, and most other spices.

## Damask Rose  *(Rosa damascena)*

**Application**  Any, especially massage and perfumes

**Note**  Base, grounding, floral

**Background**  It takes 30 flowers to make one precious drop of rose essential oil. Damask rose essential oil (attar of roses) is preferred to other rose essential oils for perfumes and beauty preparations. The damask rose blooms for only a couple of weeks—a sweet, short time. It is native to the Orient, cultivated in Bulgaria and Turkey, and it grows wild in France. It has a deep, sweet, floral, spicy scent. Since it is costly and is in so much demand, adulteration is common, so watch out. There are over 10,000 varieties of the rose. Hybrids are never used therapeutically. Legend says that all roses were white until Aphrodite, the goddess of love, pricked her foot on a thorn.

**Use**  Rose oil is an important nervine for those who feel a lack of love. A cooling tonic for the mind, it is an antidepressant and sedative for the nerves. It regulates appetite and aids in impotence and frigidity (studies point to its even being able to increase sperm count). It promotes feelings of well-being and happiness and is helpful in calming domestic strife. Uplifting and balancing, it eases grief, jealousy, and the loss of love, and is good for low self-esteem. Jeanne Rose, aromaherbalist, uses it for children in pain or grief, since it is gentle yet effective. It has been called the flower of love, a confidence builder. Although it is very expensive, it is so powerful that a small amount is effective. It is also good for dry skin, wrinkles, broken capillaries, and other skin conditions. Add 2 drops to a bath for grief or insomnia. For a massage oil, add 8 drops to 1 fluid ounce (30 ml) of sweet almond oil.

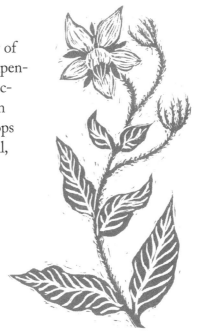

**Rose Water** Take a handful of dried rose petals, cover them with water, and bring them to a boil in an enamel pan. Simmer for 10 minutes, strain, and bottle. Keep this in the refrigerator.

**Blend** with most essential oils, especially lavender.

## Helichrysum   (*Helichrysum italicum*)
### (Also called IMMORTELLE and EVERLASTING)

**Application** Warm compresses
**Note** Base, grounding, herbaceous
**Background** Helichrysum is used as a fixative for soaps and perfumes. Native to the Mediterranean and North Africa, the plant is shrubby, with woody stems and daisylike flowers. It has an intense warm scent, honeylike with an undertone of tea scent.
**Use** Good for depression, lethargy, exhaustion, and nervous stress, this oil is grounding. It helps one accept changes, relax, and sort out problems. It has been a comfort and healer of hearts, helps increase dreams, and leads to an understanding of what hasn't been dealt with.
**Blend** with grapefruit, cypress, and neroli.

## Hyssop   (*Hyssopus officinalis*)

**Application** Bath, herb in tea
**Note** Middle, balancing, herbaceous
**Caution** Overdosing can cause convulsions. Epileptics and pregnant women should avoid it.
**Background** Hyssop has long been important in ritual, and bunches of this herb were used to sweep clean and purify ancient temples. The Greeks called it *azob* and the Hebrews *exob;* both words mean "holy herb." The essential oil

is made from the aromatic, downy, dark green leaves of this evergreen, shrub-like plant. It has a warming, bitter, pungent odor that's minty, camphorlike, and almost medicinal. It grows wild throughout America and Europe and was once used to flavor alcoholic drinks like Chartreuse and Benedictine.

**Use** If you are burned out from overwork or suffer from depression linked to grief or guilt, this essential oil works well. It helps reduce hysteria and is a nervine that clears the head and strengthens the thought processes. It is anti-inflammatory and can induce sweating. If suffering grief, melancholy, or exhaustion, add 5 to 10 drops of essential oil to the bath.

**Blend** with lavender, rosemary, myrtle, and citrus oils.

## *Sweet Marjoram* (Origanum majorana)

**Application** Inhalation; baths in moderation

**Note** Middle, balancing, herbaceous

**Caution** Overuse will knock you out. Do not give to pregnant women, the elderly, children, or those with low blood pressure.

**Background** Marjoram grows wild in the Mediterranean, Asia, France, England, Yugoslavia, and Hungary. The Greeks said that Aphrodite first cultivated this flower. Perhaps that is why they created garlands of it to crown their brides and grooms. Happiness is attributed to it, and one of its names is "joy of the mountain." Of the mint family, it has a creeping root with small, dark green leaves and tufts of purple-pink flowers, growing 1 to 3 feet (30 cm to 1 meter) tall. It has a warm, sweet, mellow, almost spicy scent. It was once planted on graves because it was believed to help the dead sleep peacefully.

**Use** Marjoram is a useful nervine for both men and women. It is very helpful in sorrow, grief, or loneliness—anytime there is emotional exhaustion. It works against insomnia and loss of appetite while comforting the heart and restoring the will to live. It is good for stress, headaches, and migraines. Since it can help a love-sick heart and decrease sexual drive, it is recommended for anyone striving to break free from an obsessive love interest.

For an aromatic bath, add 6 drops to the bathwater after the tub has filled, and swirl it around to mix. Do not soak longer than 20 minutes.

**Blend** with rosemary, lavender, and chamomile.

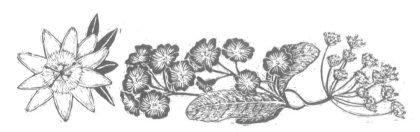

## *Myrtle*   *(Myrtus communis)*

(Also called CORSICAN PEPPER)

**Application** Most

**Note** Middle, balancing, herbaceous

**Background** Myrtle was once sacred to Aphrodite, goddess of love, beauty, and wealth. All the plants which she favored are appropriate in this chapter, because she was able to pass freely to the underworld and have access to lost loved ones. Myrtle belongs to a large family of plants that includes the bayberry, tea tree, and eucalyptus. It is a small tree with sharp, pointed leaves that grows as a garden shrub throughout Europe, the Mediterranean, and North Africa. The sweet herbal scent is similar to that of eucalyptus but not so penetrating. In the 16th century the leaves and flowers were used in the skin care lotion called angel's water. It has long been an ingredient in eau-de-colognes and toilet waters.

**Use** This mild oil is good for the elderly and children. It is a slight sedative, which helps those with self-destructive tendencies and those who are going through dark times. It has an aroma of purity and gentle cheer. Considered to bring inner wisdom, it helps the dying and those who fear death.

**Blend** with bergamot, hyssop, and clary sage.

## *Orange Blossom*   *(Citrus aurantium)*

**Application** Inhalation, bath, compress, massage

**Note** Middle, balancing, citrus

**Background** Originating in China, the orange tree is an evergreen with glossy, dark green leaves and fragrant white flowers. The oil from the bitter-orange tree is made from the blossoms. The bitter or Seville orange yields the oil called neroli. A 16th century Italian princess, Anna Maria de la Trémoille, Princess of Nerole, discovered the haunting oil and used it to scent her gloves. It is very expensive. Said to promote cell regeneration, it works well in facial creams. It has a warm, sweet, sensuous, citrus scent.

**Use** Orange should be used for shock, fear of the future, hopelessness, and depression. It is emotionally balancing and very powerful in calming emotional problems. It is helpful to those who are thin-skinned or giving up and withdrawing from life. It reduces fear of the unknown and helps get rid of feelings of emptiness, so that it is again possible to greet the days ahead with hope.

This is a great essential oil to have on hand for times of sudden emergency. Remember never to take an essential oil undiluted, and do not exceed the prescribed dosage.

**Orange Flower Water** For insomnia, shock, or uneasiness, add 2 drops of orange essential oil to 1 cup (240 ml) of water or hot herbal tea.

**Blend** with citrus oils, rosemary, and petitgrain.

## *Petitgrain* (Citrus aurantium bigaradia)
### (Also called PETITGRAIN BIGARADE)

**Application** Absorption and inhalation

**Note** Middle, balancing, citrus

**Caution** Since petitgrain can cause skin discoloration, don't go out in the sun right after application. Use no more than 3 drops in the bath.

**Background** This essential oil is a cousin to neroli and sweet-orange oils, but, because it is distilled from the leaves and twigs of the orange tree, it has a woodier and harsher scent. It is used in perfumes, colognes, foods, confections, and alcoholic drinks. The best quality essential oil comes from France.

**Use** This is an excellent oil for convalescents, for people angered from a loss, and for people who have been deeply disappointed. It is strengthening and revitalizing, good for stress and insomnia, and it enhances a state of well-being, relaxation, and balance. It leads to more open communication and helps reduce rigid thinking.

**Blend** with neroli, lemon, and jasmine.

## *Scotch Pine* (Pinus sylvestris)

**Application** Inhalation, bath

**Note** Middle, balancing, woody

**Caution** Use only 2 or 3 drops in a bath.

**Background** The fresh green scent of pine evokes the great outdoors. Pine-needle oil is safe but very powerful. Only a small amount is needed to affect the mind and body. Used by Native American Indians medicinally, this majestic tree is cultivated in the United States, Europe, and Finland.

**Use** Because this scent gives us the feeling of "breathing fresh air," it imparts a sense of life and unity, of what life is and means ultimately. It is a good restorative to use after a long illness or stress. Good for fatigue, nervous exhaustion, and tension, it acts as a stimulant, clearing the mind and lifting the spirits.

**Blend** with spicy oils, eucalyptus, and lavender.

# CHAPTER FIVE

# Shyness & Excessive Fear

*"Teach me your mood,*
*O patient stars!*
*Who climb each night*
*the ancient sky,*
*leaving on space*
*no shade, no scars,*
*no trace of age,*
*no fear to die."*

—Ralph Waldo Emerson, 1803–1882,
"The Poet"

Shyness is a very common human condition. Studies have shown that it invades every culture, with severely shy symptoms exhibited by at least 2 percent of any group—as much as 10 percent in studies in Japan. In one general study within the United States, over 80 percent of the subjects said that they had experienced shyness at one time in their lives. And it isn't a recent cultural phenomenon. Shyness is recorded in an Anglo-Saxon poem written around 1000 A.D.

What is it to be shy? Shyness can range from mild to moderate to severe (most people fall into the middle category). Mild shyness can be occasional awkwardness when speaking in public. Severe shyness can lead to full-blown anxiety attacks that make it impossible for a person to leave home. Shy people are wary in their actions and speech and shrink from self-assertion. They may be hard to approach, easily frightened by people or situations, and seemingly poised on the edge of their seats. Shyness in its moderate-to-severe form is a crippling condition of the human soul. It can be a worse handicap than physical limitations, for the shy will shrink from trying to overcome their condition.

A California social psychologist, Philip Zimbardo, undertook to understand the problems of the shy. His studies opened the door to a largely unexplored aspect of the human condition. One experiment, conducted in the early 1970s, seems to show that anyone can exhibit signs of shyness under certain situations. Students were randomly chosen to be either guards or prisoners in a mock-prison situation. What started out as a 2-week project had to be terminated within 6 days. The student guards had become cruel and misused their power, while the student prisoners were turned into wretched docile or submissive creatures who began to bow their heads and exhibit severe emotional distress.

## *Shrinking Violets & Fearful Fellows*

In 1983, Jonathon Cheek, Ph.D., author of *Conquering Shyness: The Battle Anyone Can Win*, postulated that shyness has a genetic component, a tendency that is brought out by certain conditions. Current research suggests that 15 percent of us may have this inherited tendency. Other behaviorists believe that shyness is a learned phobic reaction to social events.

Today we live in a shyness-generating society, they argue, and we often face isolation, competition, and loneliness. The shy may not learn proper social skills, they may expect themselves to perform inadequately, and, therefore, put themselves down. A child who tries to be effective in an adult-dominated world may have his efforts laughed at and be made to feel incompetent.

A racing pulse, a pounding heart, and butterflies in the stomach can signal any strong emotional reaction. For the shy, the addition of embarrassment can also cause blushing and can transform excitement into fear of these agonizing symptoms.

The picture is not entirely negative. Shyness isn't something to be stamped out, but managed. A little shyness is often admired. No one will ever say that cautious and deliberately modest people are obnoxious or overly aggressive. And most shyness is a temporary emotional reaction triggered by new people or situations. Here we present three levels of shyness and their symptoms as well as ways of managing them and learning coping skills. Essential oils chosen specifically to help certain tendencies work hand-in-hand with these management skills.

## *Degrees of Shyness*

### Mild Shyness

Many admired people, some with great accomplishments and talents, have a tendency to shyness. Some writers, scientists, and nature lovers, for example, prefer being alone. Their outward behavior does not exhibit fear, either. The mildly shy can hide their feelings. They may feel discomfort with small talk or other social functions, but they manage to cope.

The mildly shy can live with it by learning to reach out to others in small ways: smiling, offering hellos now and then to strangers, asking if co-workers need help. All these actions increase coping skills. They may volunteer their time to a worthwhile cause that interests them, such as an animal shelter, nature conservancy, garden co-op, or a center for the elderly.

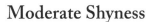

## Moderate Shyness

Most shy people fall into the middle range. Their intimidation is strong enough to disturb their social lives, causing them to avoid people and situations they fear. It is nearly impossible for them to talk openly about how they feel or to offer opinions. They blush easily and become obviously embarrassed. They are highly self-critical. The moderately shy person would like to make friends but is prevented by anxiety. Studies have shown that shy people maintain their negative self-images despite evidence of their positive qualities. They remember and repeatedly go over their humiliations but do not acknowledge their successes.

Relaxation techniques—meditation, yoga, and deep-breathing exercises—can help ease the symptoms. Visualization—practice in handling a difficult situation—has helped the performance of many athletes and can work well in shyness, too. The shy person can work at building up self-esteem, replacing negative thoughts with positive ones, and doing things for which he or she can feel a sense of accomplishment.

## Severe Shyness

The severely shy person experiences extreme dread when called on to do something in front of others, sometimes shaking, crying, and feeling overwhelmed by anxiety. At its worst, the condition becomes a severe form of neurosis that can paralyze its victim and cause deep depression and thoughts of suicide. Panic attacks and phobias are part of severe shyness. It is thought that panic attacks are caused by an accumulation of anxiety and stress, a reaction to months or years of pressure. A phobia (from the Greek *phobos*, meaning "extreme fear or terror") is a fear of natural situations or objects. It may stem from repressed anger. Both panic attacks and phobias are defenses against extreme anxiety.

Severe shyness affects its victim's life in several ways.

- It is difficult for the extremely shy person to keep or make friends or to enjoy leisure time.
- Shyness makes it hard to think clearly or communicate effectively.
- Negative feelings, like depression, anxiety, and loneliness are nearly always present.
- The very shy cannot assert themselves or express themselves, their values, and their opinions.
- Great shyness creates self-consciousness and excessive self-preoccupation.
- It sometimes leads to drug or alcohol abuse. These substances relieve the symptoms of anxiety but create more problems.

Of course, when emotions are this extreme, outside help in the form of therapy or counseling should be sought. An aromatherapy program can be followed along with conventional therapy, but make sure the physician consulted knows about it. Various organizations, like the Anxiety Disorders Association of America (ADAA) in Washington, D.C., and the National Mental Health Association in Virginia, can be contacted for help.

## Setting the Mood to Dare Not Fear

If shyness is basically fear, what does fear do to us? Our skin becomes cold and clammy. We shiver. We may have digestive problems and eating disorders. Chronic headaches may arise from psychogenic problems, such as fear and anxiety. Skin problems, like acne, boils, and other eruptions, may occur, possibly due to hormonal imbalances caused by anxiety.

The essential oils chosen for shyness are therefore warming to the body and mind, and many are very good for skin problems. Note that many of the plants either are evergreen or grow in shady, damp places. Evergreens seem to offer protection and to cleanse one of negative emotions. Shady plants seem to say, "Be humble yet calm." In any case, the essential oils listed here are calming and encourage mental strength.

## Application

When you feel cold fear settle upon you before a stress-filled event like a date, speaking engagement, or group activity, turn to the shyness-banishing essential oils. Since they are so very good in skin preparations, we include the use of scented lotions as well as other methods.

## Inhalation & Absorption

### *Lotions, Colognes & Perfumes*

Scented lotions can be inhaled at the same time that they are absorbed through the skin, thus acting in two ways at once. Below, we give directions for making your own lotion. We follow these with recipes for a perfume and a cologne you can apply whenever you need an added boost. If you make both the lotion and the perfume (or cologne), you can harmonize them by using the same scent or blend in both.

### *Cool Lotions for the Calm & Collected*

Choose a scent or a blend. Men may prefer the piney-citrus odors, women the sweeter florals. Make sure your chosen essential oils are safe for skin absorption, and choose appropriately for oily or dry skin. You can apply the lotion to your whole body and your face, taking care to avoid sensitive areas like eyes, underarms, and genitals.

### *Quick & Easy Lotion*

Purchase an unscented lotion. To 8 fluid ounces (1 cup, or 240 ml) of it, add 80 to 100 drops of essential oil (or a blend of 40 drops of one scent, 20 drops of another, and 20 drops of a third). Mix well.

### *Special Homemade Lotion*

Melt 1 to 2 tablespoons (15–30 ml) of beeswax over low heat (the more beeswax you add, the stiffer the lotion will be). Remove it from the heat. Stir in 1 cup (240 ml) of jojoba oil. Beat well and let it cool, then add 80 to 100 drops of blended essential oils. When the lotion is thick and creamy, pour it into a small glass container with a tight lid. A small jelly jar with a screw top works well. Since jojoba is chemically similar to the oils secreted by the skin, it is not oily. It absorbs well and has a long shelf life.

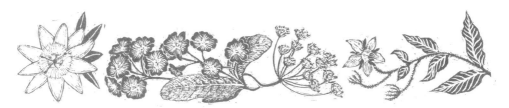

*Perfumes & Colognes*

Perfume for the Daring Woman and Cologne for the Confident Man are just two of many perfume and cologne recipes you can blend yourself. Choose one of these blends or make up your own, using your favorite essential oils. In each recipe, you'll add 48 drops of essential oil to 2 fluid ounces (¼ cup, or 60 ml) of vodka. (Castor oil is not counted in the total drops of essential oil for these recipes.)

### Perfume for the Daring Woman

*2 fluid ounces (¼ cup, or 60 ml) of vodka*
*5 drops of castor oil*
*25 drops of vanilla essential oil*
*18 drops of angelica essential oil*
*5 drops of galbanum essential oil*

Blend the ingredients and allow the mixture to steep for 2 weeks. Use the perfume in a spray atomizer.

### Cologne for the Confident Man

*¼ cup (2 fl oz, or 60 ml) of vodka*
*5 drops of castor oil*
*28 drops of rosemary essential oil*
*15 drops of juniper essential oil*
*5 drops of grapefruit essential oil*
*⅛ cup (1 fl oz, or 30 ml) lavender tea or infusion*

Make a strong lavender-bud tea or infusion; strain. Add other ingredients and blend. Allow 2 weeks to steep. Pour cologne into tightly capped bottle.

## Ingestion

*Tinctures*

At particularly stressful times, or when you want to work in depth at getting rid of your fears, you may want to try a small amount of a tincture. Both borage and gotu kola work well. When taking the tincture, you may use your perfume or cologne once a day, but don't apply the lotion. Remember, it doesn't take much to create powerful changes in the emotions, and if you overdo, you may get the opposite effect from the one desired.

   To make a tincture, put a handful of borage or gotu kola in a quart jar (or liter jar) and cover it with vodka. (Use about 1 ounce of dried or fresh herb to 1 quart of vodka.) Place it in a sunny window for 2 weeks, strain, and store.

### Borage  (Borago officinalis)

Borage "always brings courage," said the herbalist John Gerard in 1597. In 1699 John Evelyn claimed that borage was "of known virtue to revive the hypochondriac and cheer the hard student."

It increases vitality by stimulating the adrenal glands to produce epinephrine, which gears the body up for action. It brings on perspiration and relieves irritable-bowel syndrome. This annual, easily grown in filtered shade, has a pleasant cucumber taste. Use the fleshy, coarse leaves and flowers. For fear, depression, anxiety, or sadness, take the tincture, 1 dropperful (20 drops, or 1 ml) three times a day, until symptoms subside.

### Gotu Kola  (Centella asiatica)

This herb grows in tropical and subtropical river valleys in central China, India, and Africa. It was used in ayurvedic medicine to promote mental calm and clarity. It is an energizer, nerve tonic, and brain tonic. Himalayan yogis and Taoist hermits take it for longevity, and research indicates that it retards the aging process by its ability to revitalize brain cells and promote cellular repair. It is even said to help in schizophrenia and other mental disorders by balancing the left and right hemispheres of the brain. It is also used in meditation. This tender perennial likes humidity and filtered sun. Use the leaves and stalks. Take 2 teaspoons (10 ml) of the tincture twice a day.

**Caution**  Don't exceed the recommended dosage, since it can have a narcotic effect.

## Bach Flower Remedies

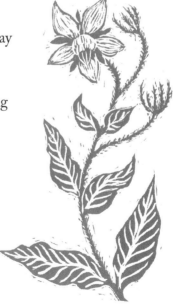

For shyness, take these flower essences, 4 drops a day under the tongue.

**Aspen**  vague, unfounded fears, apprehension

**Centaury**  self-denial, difficulty in saying no, feeling easily exploited

**Larch**  lack of self-confidence, failure to try

**Mimulus**  phobias, e.g., fear of the dark, public speaking, heights, growing old, and being alone

**Rockrose**  fright, terror, e.g., in sudden emergency

**Water Violet**  aloofness and unapproachability on the part of loners whom others find remote and difficult to befriend

# Daring Essential Oils

## *Angelica*    *(Angelica archangelica)*

**Application**  Skin creams, bath, massage, inhalation
**Note**  Top, uplifting, herbaceous
**Caution**  The essential oil is not for use by pregnant women or diabetics. It can cause sun sensitivity.
**Background**  In China angelica is used to fortify the spirit. In Europe it has a long medicinal history. The plant loves wet, cool, shady places and has a rich, spicy, yet earthy scent. It is used in beauty products, especially for the skin, because of its soothing quality. The liqueur Benedictine gets its flavor from this tall biennial plant. The roots and stalk were candied and traditionally used to improve energy levels.
**Use**  Like many of the essential oils in this chapter, angelica is warming. It takes away fear, phobias, timidity, shyness, and indecision and replaces them with relaxation and a sense of reality. It is good for the weak, timid, fearful, and hopeless and for those who lack perseverance. It is refreshing. It reduces weakness, nausea, anorexia, migraine, nervous tension, and stress-related disorders. This essential oil bestows strength and the courage to stick with things.
**Blend** with patchouli, clary sage, and citrus oils.

## *Galbanum*    *(Ferula galbaniflua)*

**Application**  Inhalation, massage, skin lotions
**Background**  This essential oil is now distilled in Europe and the United States and used as a fixative in perfumes. In Lebanon it was once considered an aphrodisiac. Ancient civilizations found it an enlightening incense, and in Egypt it was an ingredient in embalming and perfumes. It has a green, yet woody, pine scent, somewhat spicy. A large perennial plant, its stems exude a milky juice or resin that is collected through incisions at the stem base.
**Use**  Galbanum creates calm and balance. It is good for people on the edge of fear, tension, hysteria, or paranoia, as it eases rigidity and helps one go with the flow. It aids in cases of acne, boils, and other skin problems.
**Blend** with violet, geranium, lavender, and pine scents.

# *Grapefruit* *(Citrus paradisi)*

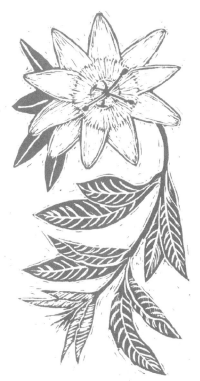

**Application** Inhalation, in a diffuser; massage, lotions

**Note** Top, uplifting, citrus

**Caution** Use it sparingly in bath or skin oils, as it is powerful. It has a short shelf life.

**Background** The grapefruit is a cultivated tree with glossy dark green leaves and the familiar large yellow fruit. The essential oil is distilled in the United States by cold-pressing the fruit.

**Use** Grapefruit has a balancing, uplifting scent, like all citrus essential oils. It is especially good for performance anxiety and helps in cases of fearfulness or stress. It regulates the appetite and is helpful for migraines. It also helps oily skin, acne, and cellulite. The grapefruit's odor stimulates neurotransmitters that tend to make a person feel more hopeful in the face of self-doubt and overwhelming events. It promotes well-being, positive thinking, and a zest for life.

**Blend** with lemon, orange blossom, and rosemary.

# *Juniper* *(Juniperus communis)*

**Application** Inhalation, massage, bath

**Note** Middle, balancing, resinous

**Caution** Avoid it if you are pregnant or have kidney problems.

**Background** Juniper is an evergreen shrub or tree with stiff needles. Its scent is light, bittersweet, warming, and turpentinelike. An embalming herb in ancient Egypt, it has been burned in temples and associated with ritual cleansing because of its powerful detoxifying properties. In European folk medicine, the oil, which comes from the berries, was regarded as a cure-all. The tree was believed to surround one with protective energy.

**Use** This nervine helps banish lassitude and languor and fosters alertness and positive thinking. It clears and rejuvenates the mind, removing weakness and flushing out unwanted emotions. Take it when you need to feel centered, balanced, and uplifted. It is also very good for oily skin, acne, and cellulite. Add 5 drops to the bath or to a diffuser.

**Blend** with bergamot, sandalwood, and rosemary.

## *Peru Balsam*   (Myroxylon balsamum)

**Application**  Inhalation, skin preparations

**Background**  Peru balsam is a large tropical tree with fragrant flowers and resinous juice. It has a sweet balsamic scent, with a vanillalike undertone. In Central America it is used in many medicinal preparations and as a fixative in lotions and perfumes.

**Use**  Stimulating, warming, opening, and comforting, this oil is good to use for tension, stress, and fear of new situations. Studies show it promotes the growth of skin cells, and it is used for dry, chapped skin and other skin problems.

**Blend** with spices, rose, and petitgrain.


## *Rosemary*   (Rosmarinus officinalis)

**Application**  Inhalation, bath

**Note**  Middle, balancing, herbaceous

**Caution**  Avoid it in cases of pregnancy, high blood pressure, and epilepsy.

**Background**  Rosemary ("dew of the sea") was said to bring luck, and early herbalists believed that wearing a sprig of it could cure nervous ailments. It is a tender perennial, evergreen shrub with fat needle-pointed leaves that grows in partial shade and has a piney, misty scent. Sir Thomas Moore said it was "the herb sacred to remembrance and therefore to friendship." John Gerard said it "comforteth the heart and maketh it merry." It is a great detoxicant and one of the first herbs used in food preparation. It is well-loved in England and originates in the Mediterranean. The flowering tops and needles are used.

**Use**  Studies show it stimulates the adrenal cortex. It is an energizer, clearing the mind and helping with mental fatigue and memory. A great nervous-system balancer as well as tonic, it helps relieve tension and gives strength to the faint-hearted. Uplifting and invigorating, it warms the body and spirit, dispelling sadness and headaches. It is listed in the *British Herbal Pharmacopoeia* for depressive states with debility or weakness. Good for stress and mood swings, it can help someone who is trying to learn to build on existing relationships, face what is feared, and keep from being defensive.

For a bath, use 10 drops. To make a rub for the forehead, add 1 to 2 drops to 1 fluid ounce (30 ml) of sunflower oil.

**Blend** with basil, frankincense, and cedarwood.

# *Spruce*    *(Picea mariana)*

**Application**  Skin lotions, inhalation
**Note**  Middle, balancing, woody
**Background**  This evergreen, with its refreshing outdoor aroma, grows wild in Canada and Europe. It is one species from the large family of pines and is valuable medicinally. Make sure you get the true spruce essential oil.
**Use**  Spruce oil is detoxifying and helps heal wounds and ulcers. It calms anxiety and stress, and it is very helpful to the nervous system. It awakens self-confidence, patience, courage, and strength.
**Blend** with angelica, lemon, and mint.

# *Vanilla*    *(Vanilla planifolia)*

**Application**  Creams, body lotions, bath, inhalation
**Note**  Middle, balancing, resinous
**Background**  Make sure you obtain the true vanilla essential oil. It is widely adulterated, and much of the vanilla extract (or tincture) sold in grocery stores is imitation. The vanilla vines grow in Central America and the West Indies. The vanilla beans have no aroma until dried. After drying, the outside of the bean may have white crystals. This is the *vanillin,* from which come the familiar flavor and aroma. In Mexico there are hummingbirds that pollinate the vine, but elsewhere, pollination is done completely by hand, a time-consuming job. Vanilla is used in tincture form to flavor cookies, cakes, and ice cream. The characteristic scent is soft and sweet.
**Use**  Vanilla mildly stimulates one to make an extra effort. It warms, calms, and relaxes, softening frustration and irritability. It revitalizes the body and helps make one attractive to others.
**Blend** with sandalwood, vetiver, and other spicy scents.

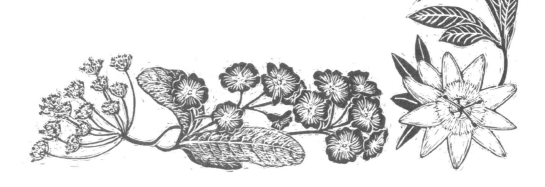

# *V i o l e t*  (*Viola odorata*)

### (Also called SWEET VIOLET)

**Application**  Syrup; leaf absolute in inhalation

**Note**  Top, uplifting, floral

**Background**  This modest flower, which hides in damp, shady places, is native to Europe and is cultivated in gardens worldwide. Both the flower and the leaf have long held a place in herbal medicine. Violets have been used in love potions, perfumes, confections, and flavorings. The flowers make "syrup of violet." Pliny said it helped dizziness, while Homer claimed it regulated the anger of Athenian citizens. In 1762 a German physician, Bezaar Zimmermann, claimed violet was an astonishing aphrodisiac, while other doctors said it was a stimulating tonic that could turn a dullard into the life of the party. It is a tender plant with heart-shaped leaves and fragrant blue flowers. It has a strong, leafy aroma with floral undertones.

**Use**  The scent is believed to comfort and strengthen the heart. Violet is a stimulant and helps with headaches, insomnia, and nervous exhaustion. The syrup is considered a mild painkiller because it contains salicylic acid, as does aspirin. Violet is good for the skin, particularly acne and large pores. Helpful to the mildly reticent, it is gentle enough for the elderly and children over 2 years of age.

**Syrup of Violet**  Pour 1 cup (240 ml) of boiling water over a handful of leaves and flowers. Steep covered for 6 minutes, then strain. Add equal amounts of honey, and mix well. Store this in the refrigerator. Take 1 teaspoon (5 ml) as needed up to three times a day.

**Blend** with tuberose, hops, and basil.

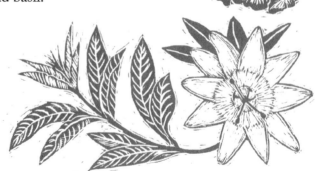

# CHAPTER SIX

# Bad Temper & Anger

*"Why should there be
such turmoil
and such strife,
to spin in length
this feeble line of life?"*

—Francis Bacon, 1561–1626,
translation of Psalm 90

Anger is one of our most primitive emotions, arising from deep in the "old brain." It is a leftover survival emotion, a weapon in the old competition for the best mate, the best food, the best territory. To paraphrase Sigmund Freud, anger is a tool we use when something threatens to prevent us from reaching a goal. When we are frustrated, we feel angry, and we vent our anger in an effort to remove the frustration. Our aggressive displays are meant to cause doubt, fear, or humiliation, so that whoever or whatever is blocking us backs down or goes away. We can be angry at people, things, situations, and even ourselves.

## Causes of Anger

Many psychiatrists and psychologists feel that our aggressive behavior is always traceable to something that has been denied us. What do we get angry about? We swear and slap our hands on the steering wheel because some driver cuts ahead of us to steal our parking space. The child who is told "No candy" at the grocery screams and stamps his foot. We blow up at a lover who tells us to get lost. We are furious when the boss makes unreasonable demands that cut into our leisure time. All these situations are instances of desire denied.

Primitive humans, it would seem, had it relatively easy emotionally. All they had to worry about was food, shelter, and procreation. Their anger stemmed from denial of any of these three basic needs. And they could express their feelings forcefully and directly. Today, however, our lives are quite diverse and complex. We face confusion and uncertainty. It is a frustrating society, with massive disregard for individuals and individual needs. Look at the broad range of problems related to anger and aggression: murder, bombings, riots, arson, gang fights, domestic violence, child abuse. We have created a society of violence because we have failed to recognize anger as an intrinsic part of ourselves. Our lack of understanding has made it impossible to get the anger under control.

## Internalized Anger

Because anger is not a socially acceptable emotion, we grow up learning to internalize it. Often we are more angry internally than externally. We are so good at hiding our anger that we can be seething inside while telling ourselves that we are calm. Held-in frustrations and resentments can create an imbalance in the body. Unexpressed anger can not only warp the personality but can manifest itself in physical problems.

### Temper, Temper

Think about it. When we are angry, our faces turn red, our breathing quickens, our blood pressure goes up, and we say, "I feel like I'm going to explode." We want to scream and strike out, our hands shake, we feel hot and sweaty, we "see red." Now, what if we suppress those feelings? Doesn't it make sense that eventually we would develop headaches, stomachaches, dizziness, tiredness, even severe irrational behavior and self-defeating neuroses? In *Coping with Anger* Paul J. Gelinos states: "In many years as a clinical psychologist working with young adults, I cannot recall a single case of neurosis or emotional disturbance that did not have unresolved anger as the main overt or intrinsic element in the disorder."

It is hard to function as a child in the big adult world. Children between the ages of 1 and 5 often have temper tantrums. Sometimes they are frustrated at being unable to communicate their feelings or desires. Sometimes their feelings and desires are discounted because they are young. Teenagers show anger through withdrawal, moodiness, rebellion, and aggressive acts. They must be shown how to set and reach attainable goals for themselves and be given time to talk out their confused ideas and feelings. Adults may be short-fused and have outbursts of anger. The elderly may be manipulative and demanding.

62

Anger is a powerful emotion. Trying to do away with it or stuffing it back inside ourselves won't work. Anger will always be a part of our lives. We have to learn how to deal with it. We must learn to express our feelings effectively, not allow them to feed the monster of anger. We must find a way to control our emotional displays, so that no one gets hurt.

## Uses of Anger

Anger is a signal. It can act for our own good. It lets us know that we have an unmet need and urges us to figure out what that need is and to do something about it. It spurs us on to conquer the frustrations that have blocked our path.

We have to find out what has caused our anger. Often the event that triggers an angry outburst isn't the root of it at all. For instance, the child who punches a friend on the playground is in fact angry because of his parents' divorce. A husband who is angry at being passed over for promotion takes it out in a meaningless argument with his wife. We have all become masters at hiding what is really bothering us.

Before we can analyze the situation, we have to calm down. We may count to 10, take deep breaths, or go for a walk. Then we may be ready to try to look at the problem clearly and pinpoint what's wrong. At this point the essential oils can help.

## Setting the Mood for Soothing Anger

How can the essential oils temper an angry mood? They can aid the body to rebalance itself and cool hot feelings. They can help dispel the physical manifestations of long-held anger: headaches, touchiness, irritability, and exhaustion. They can regulate, too, so that the degree of frustration is not out of line with the situation at hand. Once a person has calmed down enough to be in touch with his or her true feelings and to express them clearly, he will feel the relief of being in control. The frustrations will still be there, but they can be dealt with.

## Application

Many of the essential oils in this chapter are best used in inhalation and are especially good for lung and bronchial problems. Remember, anger at once changes the breathing pattern. These essential oils also have been used traditionally to enhance meditation and are especially suited to work on the inner self. More than one comes from the pine family. The pines are very good at cooling and calming a fiery temperament.

Another factor in anger is digestive upset. Constant battle with aggressive tendencies tends to cause ulcers, diverticulitis, acid stomach, and the like. The herbs suggested for tinctures (under Ingestion) aid digestion.

Choose an appropriate time to administer your anger-soothing "potion." For sudden angry flare-ups, have a prepared remedy on hand. Use it for those moments when anger is inappropriate or threatens to spoil an important occasion. A planned daily program of therapy for chronic anger is best carried out in the morning hours. This starts the day off on the right foot. Additional treatment can be given later in the day, if needed. Expect therapy for deep-seated anger to last at least 2 weeks. It takes some time for a person to find new ways of dealing with problems.

Do NOT use the inhalation and tincture methods together, since that would constitute overdosage and might cause increased irritability. If you choose inhalation, you can inhale a few drops from a handkerchief at times during the day and then use a diffuser or vaporizer in the evening. Try it for a week. If you notice a difference, discontinue the treatment until it is needed again. If you see no change, give yourself a 3-day rest. Resume for another week, if you need it.

Herbal tinctures are especially good for the more deep-seated problems (see Ingestion below).

The Bach flower remedies can be used in conjunction with either inhalation or a tincture or on their own.

## Inhalation

For a quick fix, put 4 to 6 drops of essential oil in a bowl of hot water. Close your eyes, and inhale the steam for 5 minutes.

When you are going out of the house, apply several drops to a handkerchief and put it in a plastic bag. Inhale from it when you feel the need: 5 minutes at a time for adults (12 years old and older) and 1 to 2 minutes at a time for children (use essential oils especially suited to children).

At home on the weekend or in the evening, add 4 to 6 drops to a humidifier or steam vaporizer. Run it for about an hour.

## Ingestion

### Herb Vinegar Tinctures

Vinegar tinctures can be administered to children, the elderly, and those adults who do not wish to consume alcohol. Make tinctures from the following herbs by using 1 cup (240 ml) of fresh material or ½ cup (120 ml) of dried to 2 cups (480 ml) of a good apple cider vinegar with an acidity level of at least 5 percent. Steep for 2 weeks and strain.

**Caution** These recipes call for use of the herb (flowers, leaves, etc.). DO NOT use the essential oil when making these tinctures.

## *Chrysanthemum (Chrysanthemum morifolium)*

Use the flowers. They make a bittersweet and tangy-tasting tincture that is a tonic and diuretic and lowers blood pressure. The Chinese say that it clears "liver heat," i.e., it cools a hot-headed person. It is balancing and removes headaches.

This perennial flower grows wild in many parts of China and is considered the flower of immortality. Cultivation of it began 2,000 years ago. Tea from these flowers was served to Chinese emperors. It is the emblem of Japan and was brought to the United States in 1798. It grows in sun or partial shade.

**Tincture** Use the flower petals. Take 1 teaspoon (5 ml) of the tincture in 1 cup (240 ml) of cool water up to three times a day.

## *St.-John's-Wort (Hypericum perforatum)*

Use the leaves and flowers. This is a bittersweet herb with cooling properties. It helps the elderly deal with anger when feeling lonely or cast aside. It bolsters feelings of self-worth in adults. It is not for children under 6, but children from 6 to 12 will benefit from the reduced dosage if they are angry about divorce, death, or adjustment to new surroundings. It has a good flavor and improves digestion. It has been called an energy booster, yet is also a sedative, restoring balance to the nervous system. Good for irritability, it lightens the mood, deals with emotional disorders and depressive tendencies, and improves concentration. Herbalists say that a tincture taken twice a day for several months will produce profound changes on a deep level. Some change should be noticeable within 2 weeks. The tincture must be red to be effective. Researchers have found that it increases neurotransmitter function in the brain.

This plant was used to treat wounds during the Crusades. It grows in shady woods, meadows, and roadsides and has beautiful yellow flowers.

**Caution** St. John's-wort can cause sun sensitivity.

**Tincture** Use the leaves and flowers (fresh or dried). Make sure the tincture is a deep red color. If it is not strong enough, strain it and add more plant material. Let it steep for another 2 weeks. For irritability and nerves, persons 12 and over may take 1 to 2 eyedroppersful (20–40 drops, or 1–2 ml) two to three times a day. Give children 5 to 10 drops under the tongue. Take this for up to 2 months, then give the body a rest, resuming if necessary.

### Self-Heal  (Prunella vulgaris)

This herb is another good one for balancing energy, cooling angry flare-ups, and bringing the body back to normal. Slightly bitter, it is good for digestive complaints and headaches since it is a natural painkiller. The Chinese consider it cooling for "liver fire" in persons who are overly irritable, angry, or excitable, or who have high blood pressure. The plant is a small, low creeping herb with hairy stems and purplish blue flowers, found in woodlands and fields. It is a member of the mint family.

**Tincture**  Use the flower spikes and leaves. The dosage is 1 teaspoon (5 ml) every morning for persons 12 and older, or ¼ teaspoon (1 ml) for children, for up to 1 week. Discontinue for 3 days, and resume if necessary.

### Spikenard  (Nardostachys jatamansi)

This tender aromatic herb grows 3 to 6 feet (1 to 3 meters) tall and has large leaves, small clustered flowers, and a pungent root. It is mentioned in the Bible and was used in ancient Rome to make perfume. It grows wild in the mountainous regions of India, China, and Japan.

**Caution**  Pregnant women should avoid spikenard.

**Tincture**  Put ½ ounce (14 g) of powdered root in 1 pint (2 cups, or 480 ml) of vinegar. Heat gently for 10 minutes. Let it sit in a sealed jar for 7 to 10 days. Strain. Take it in the mornings. Persons 12 years of age and older: 1 teaspoon (5 ml) in juice. The elderly, frail, or children 6 to 12: ½ teaspoon (2.5 ml) in juice. Children 2 to 6 years old: ¼ teaspoon (1 ml) in juice.

**Vinegar Syrup**  Make the vinegar tincture, adding to it 1 ounce (28 g) of dried spearmint. After straining, add equal amounts of honey or pure maple syrup, and heat to blend the mixture. Cool and bottle. Children enjoy this sweet syrup, and it can be kept for 6 months. Person 12 years old and older: 1 teaspoon (5 ml). The elderly, frail, or children 6 to 12: ½ teaspoon (2.5 ml).

Use the tincture to help end bad behavior and moodiness. Use the syrup to help calm hyperactivity, bad behavior, and grumpiness. Stop when a change is noticeable. Administer for no more than 1 week without a break of 3 days.

## Bach Flower Remedies

I recommend these flower remedies, 4 drops under the tongue, as needed or twice a day.

66

**Holly** Use for hatred, jealousy, or envy stemming from a strong desire for more love. Suffering, often with no real cause.

**Vine** For the confident, capable, self-assured born leaders who are often thought to be demanding and domineering.

**Walnut** Aids in periods of transition and adjustment, e.g., a divorce, a new job, a move; need for protection against peer pressure and other people's negativity.

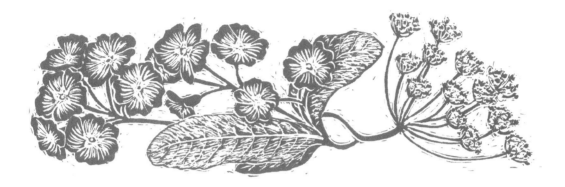

# *Soothing Essential Oils*

## *Himalayan Cedar* *(Cedrus deodara)*

### (Also called DEODAR)

**Application** Inhalation

**Note** Base, grounding, woody

**Caution** Do not take this if you are pregnant. It can irritate sensitive skin.

**Background** The reddish brown wood comes from a majestic tree that originated in India and grows at altitudes of 4,000 to 6,000 feet. The ancient Egyptians used the oil in embalming and associated its scent with the safe passage of the soul to the next world. Eastern medicine used it for bronchial infections. For centuries, the cedars of the mountains of Lebanon *(Cedrus libani)* were visited as a holy shrine. Cedar is widely used in incense, and the wood, whose camphorlike scent repels insects, was used to build temples.

**Use** This oil releases aggression caused by fear or anger. Cooling to the senses, relaxing, and sedating, it is nevertheless stimulating. It imparts harmony, helps the mind to analyze, helps with feelings of disconnection, and rejuvenates the life forces. It enhances awareness and promotes spirituality, balance, poise, calm, and control. In meditation, it is very good to use when trying to link up with one's inner self.

**Blend** with rosewood, neroli, and jasmine.

## Fir Balsam *(Abies balsamea)*

### (Also called CANADA BALSAM)

**Application** Inhalation, in a diffuser; sparingly in ointments and lotions

**Note** Middle, balancing, woody

**Caution** Do not use this in large doses.

**Background** Fir balsam has a sweet, soft, piney and fruity scent. The small pyramidal tree grows wild in European forests and has been planted in gardens worldwide. Oils are made from a number of varieties of evergreen tree, and their properties differ, so it is important to know which oil to ask for. Fir balsam oil has been used internally by North American Indians in rituals and externally for cuts and sores.

**Use** The warming quality of this essential oil is good for anger connected with depression. It releases tension, is stimulating yet relaxing, and is cleansing, calming, and balancing. Very refreshing to breathe, it is good for all chest, lung, and bronchial problems.

**Blend** with woody scents and lavender.

## Hemlock Spruce *(Tsuga canadensis)*

**Application** Inhalation, bath

**Note** Middle, balancing, woody

**Background** This large evergreen tree has slender branches and small brown cones. Native to the east coast of the United States, it grows mainly in Vermont, Virginia, and New York. Widely used in room sprays, detergents, and bath and toiletry items, it has a pleasing, fresh, fruity-sweet, balsamic scent.

**Use** A warming, refreshing tonic and nervine, it is good for deeply seated anger or aggression stemming from depression. It is calming, good for tension and stress. It is a great balancer, uplifting as well as grounding, imparting feelings of social stability, strength, understanding, and self-worth. It is a good scent for meditation or yoga, opening one up to inner spirituality. It is good for physical problems of a respiratory nature.

**Blend** with galbanum, rosemary, and lavender.

# *Lemongrass*   *(Cymbopogon citratus)*

**Application**  Inhalation, skin care, bath products

**Note**  Top, uplifting, herbaceous

**Caution**  Lemongrass can irritate sensitive skin. Don't confuse it with lemon verbena oil.

**Background**  This fast-growing, tall perennial grass, native to Asia, has long been used in Indian medicine for infections and fevers. It is in demand worldwide for perfumes, flavoring, soaps, and skin-care products. Cultivated mainly in South India, it is considered very healing. The herb is used widely in Asian, Mexican, and South American cookery and has proved to be very good for digestion and digestive upsets. It has a strong lemon scent with a grassy undertone.

**Use**  It communicates sunshine! A cheerful pick-me-up, refreshing, invigorating, and revitalizing, it is a stimulating tonic and nervine that calms the nervous system, eases stress, and ameliorates headaches. It creates an awareness of self and helps one deal with the unpredictable events of life and the twists and turns of fate. It is especially good for grumpy morning persons and those who have trouble concentrating in the morning. Research from India shows that it acts as a sedative on the central nervous system. It is cooling, and it aids in respiratory problems.

**Blend** with basil, jasmine, and lavender.


# *Spearmint*   *(Mentha spicata)*

**Application**  Inhalation, in diffuser; herb in tincture

**Note**  Top, uplifting, herbaceous

**Caution**  Avoid spearmint during pregnancy. Dilute it heavily for absorption since it is powerful (no more than 3 drops in a bath). Do not give it to babies under 2. Do not use for more than 1 week without a 3-day break.

**Background**  The mint family is well known to us through its use in flavoring toothpastes, mouthwashes, foods, and drinks. Spearmint is similar to peppermint but much milder, with sharp-pointed, lance-shaped leaves and pink or pale-violet flowers. Its odor and flavor are warm, spicy, and minty. It grows prolifically and is widely cultivated in Russia, the United States, Spain, and the Mediterranean. The ancient Greeks used it as a restorative in baths. Spearmint is good for digestive problems, stomachaches, and for the respiratory system. It helps asthma and lung congestion. The flowers, leaves, and stems are used.

**Use**  It is good for hyperactive children, especially if all soft drinks are removed from their diet. It stimulates the mind, raises the spirits, uplifts and lightens dark moods, and helps ease strain and tension. Pleasant and cooling, it is a nervine and tonic for hotheads. Refreshing, comforting, and anesthetic, it soothes and lightens foul tempers. It has been said to make one feel young again. For headaches, a massage oil can be made (12 to 15 drops of essential oil per fluid ounce of carrier oil) and rubbed into the temples.

**Blend** with jasmine, rosemary, and basil.

## *Sweet Orange*   *(Citrus sinensis dulcis)*

**Application**  Inhalation, in diffuser; lotion, bath

**Note**  Top, uplifting, citrus

**Caution**  This oil is very powerful. Use it in low dosages (3 drops in a bath) and give very low dosages to children, for short periods only.

**Background**  The orange tree is an evergreen, native to China and cultivated in Brazil, the United States, and the Mediterranean. The sweet orange peel tincture is used to flavor pharmaceuticals, because adults and children alike love the taste. It is used in soaps and perfumes. The Chinese find it a good medicinal that calms digestive upsets and increases bronchial secretions. It has a pleasing citrus scent, sharper than neroli.

**Use**  This sweet, radiant oil seems to bring along sunshine. It burns out anger, calms nervous uneasiness, and encourages joy and laughter. It is a sedative, yet stimulates energy, and is refreshing, cooling, and opening. Sweet orange tends to decrease blood pressure. It is antidepressive and mildly hypnotic.

**Blend** with neroli, clary sage, and spicy oils.

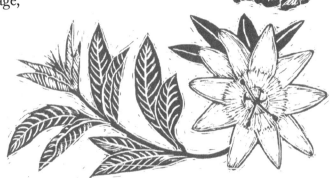

70

# CHAPTER SEVEN

# Stress, Worry & Anxiety

*"Better never trouble trouble
until trouble troubles you;
for you only make your trouble
double-trouble when you do."*

—David Keppel, b. 1846, "Trouble"

Stress is a major threat to health. Medical specialists have blamed stress for a wide range of ills: headaches, skin rashes, heart disease, high blood pressure, heart attacks, backaches, stomach and intestinal disorders, sexual dysfunction, chronic depression, and mental debility. The American Academy of Family Physicians has estimated that nearly two-thirds of all trips to the family doctor are for stress-related symptoms. Recently the National Mental Health Association put that figure up to 75 to 90 percent. What, then, is stress?

We become "stressed-out" when we feel overburdened or overwhelmed by events. A long-term, chronic situation like a family conflict may be stressful; so may a short-term problem that goes away in days or hours. How much stress a person can take is an individual matter. A deadline at work may invigorate and challenge Martha, say, but cause Annie to collapse in despair. But let's say that Martha is faced with a long, drawn-out, and bitter divorce. As the days and months drag on, she feels the wear and tear on her emotional self. When the boss throws her a project that has a pressing deadline, Martha is overwhelmed.

Life is a series of ups and downs, and we've all experienced stress at one time or another. Stress isn't all bad. A certain amount of stress gears us up to do the best we can; it keeps us in top form. To live and grow we must experience change. According to studies done in the 1960s by stress researchers Thomas Holmes and Richard Rahe, change is stressful whether it is change for the better or for the worse. Most often, stress becomes a problem when we are confronted with big changes or challenges over long periods of time. It is then that we become overanxious, tired, and burned out. A study at the University of California at Berkeley indicates that everyday stress—not the big challenges—

71

may be the greatest contributor to stress overload: irritating noise, a grumpy neighbor, a rowdy teenager, housework, or too many responsibilities.

## Signs of Stress

When we feel stress, the fight-or-flight response kicks in. This primitive response prepares us to handle emergencies: either to fight back or to run. In our modern world, we handle things less directly. If you chew the boss out, you could lose your job. And you can't run off and leave your demanding teenagers. So you hold everything in, and your system goes into overload. When the fight-or-flight signals are set off, the body responds by sending out signals to the adrenal glands. The adrenal glands secrete neurochemicals that ready the body for action by increasing heart rate, breathing, alertness, and muscle response. One of them, *epinephrine,* is a hormone geared to boost energy. Worry, the mental response to stress, triggers the brain to release another powerful hormone, *cortisol* (hydrocortisone). This hormone speeds up the metabolism.

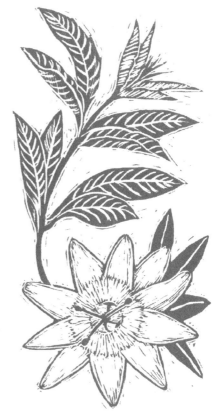

What if these hormones are summoned but not used? The body is then additionally stressed by an overabundance of energy. The glands become weakened, and the body's balance is upset. The immune system itself becomes suppressed from fighting to keep the adrenal glands going. This can be a deadly cycle, for once the immune system is damaged, the body is open to assault from all kinds of disease.

We'd all like to banish stress without changing our workloads or our busy life-styles. It is not impossible. What's needed is stress and anxiety management, so that the nervous system can "heal" and strengthen itself and so that the body does not reach a critical state. First, and most important, when you are entering a stressful period in your life, prepare for it. Then watch for the warning signs that tell you when you are overstressed. These can be physical or mental symptoms. Males are most likely to suffer physical symptoms, while females suffer more from mental.

72

## Physical Warning Signals

Any problems relating to the digestion, the respiratory system, or the skin (like acne, psoriasis, and rashes) can be a warning of stress overload. Some people experience one or a few of these symptoms: nausea, diarrhea, constipation, ulcers, teeth grinding, muscle spasms, lightheadedness, dizzy spells, fainting, imbalance, difficulty in breathing or a feeling of smothering or choking, palpitations, chest pain or pressure, tingling or numbness, headaches, and a feeling that everything is hazy and far away.

## Mental Warning Signals

Mental symptoms include inability to concentrate, general diminished ability, excessive anxiety, obsessions, and depression. The National Mental Health Association pamphlet "Stress: Coping with Everyday Problems" lists the danger signals of stress. Ask yourself these questions.

### *NMHA Stress Checklist*

- Do minor problems and disappointments upset you excessively?
- Do life's small pleasures fail to satisfy you?
- Do you feel unable to stop thinking about your worries?
- Do you feel inadequate or do you suffer from self-doubt?
- Do you feel constantly tired?
- Do you experience flashes of anger over minor problems?
- Do you notice a change in your sleeping or eating patterns?
- Do you suffer from chronic pain, headaches, or backaches?

If you answered yes to most of these questions, and if you feel your life has gotten out of control, consider talking to someone—a friend, spouse, doctor, spiritual advisor, or someone at your local mental health association. The American Institute of Stress in Yonkers, New York, may offer more information.

When you realize you are suffering from stress, you can take action. Management includes relaxation techniques as well as the use of essential oils to modify the body's response. Relaxation triggers changes in the nervous and endocrine systems: breathing slows down, and blood pressure becomes lower. Aromatherapy can then act to reverse the stress damage.

## Setting the Mood for a New Calm

Set aside a period for quiet reflection every day—10 to 30 minutes either in the morning, at noon, or at night. Make this a part of your routine. The time will be yours to take care of yourself, to compose your thoughts, to think of pleasant things or of nothing at all. Take the phone off the hook and lock the door, if you have to, or get up a few minutes earlier than the rest of the household. If you choose, listen to music. A recent study showed that "Nuages" and "Prelude á l'après-midi d'un faune" by Claude Debussy reduce stress reactions. You may choose any soothing music, classical or otherwise. Just don't play anything irritating or anything with lyrics that remind you of stress.

## Application

### Inhalation

During your quiet time, choose a scent for nhalation. You may want to blend the essential oils suggested in this chapter with some that are good for other conditions. For example, if stress-related depression is dragging you down, you might choose one of the essential oils listed in chapter 3. If you are troubled by sleep disturbances, you might strengthen your blend with one of the sleep-inducing essential oils from chapter 10. Try making several separate blends, each with a completely different set of scents. Use one blend for a week, then another blend for a week. This helps keep your body balanced, not overwhelmed with one scent or scent blend.

#### Scented Cotton Ball

Place 1 to 3 drops of an essential oil or a blend on a cotton ball. Inhale it for 3 to 5 minutes, breathing deeply and slowly. Keep your eyes closed and think of lovely things or listen to relaxing music. You may also take the scented cotton ball with you in a sealed plastic bag. Use it when you feel stress building up.

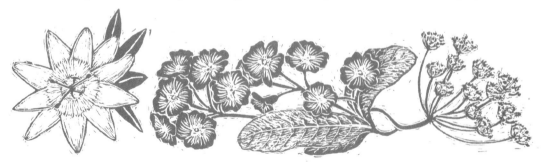

If you feel especially under stress and need a deeper therapy, you may replace the inhalation method by absorption with warm compresses or footbaths or by ingestion of herbal tea. Follow only one method of therapy at a time. These therapies can be used for up to 2 weeks. If more therapy is needed, take a break for 2 or 3 days, then resume. You may choose to alternate therapies, using absorption one day, inhalation the next.

## Absorption

### Warm Compress

Fill a small bowl with warm water, add 4 to 10 drops of an essential oil or blend, and mix well. Saturate a cotton cloth in the water, squeeze it out, and apply the compress either to the forehead (especially good for headaches—just don't let it get in the eyes) or to the abdomen (especially good for panic and exhaustion). Rewarm the cloth by dipping it back in the water. Reapply. Do this for up to 30 minutes.

### Warm Footbath

This is especially good when you are feeling chilled from being overly upset. It is very relaxing. Add 4 to 6 drops of essential oil to a small tub of warm water. Toss in a handful of Epsom salts, mix, and soak your feet for 15 to 20 minutes.

## Ingestion

### Herbal Teas

The following herbs can be used to make a relaxing cup of tea to be sipped in the evening. They can also be used instead of the essential oils in warm compresses and footbaths.

**Caution** Use the herb (flower, leaves, etc.) and NOT the essential oil for these recipes.

### Calendula  (Calendula officinalis)

The bright orange flower petals are used to make a cooling, slightly bitter-tasting tea.

**Herbal Tea** Add 2 teaspoons (10 ml) of dried or 4 teaspoons (20 ml) of fresh petals to 1 cup (240 ml) of boiling water, and steep 5 to 10 minutes. Drink twice a day as needed.

### Primrose  (Primula vulgaris) & Cowslip  (Primula veris)

Primrose and cowslip are members of the same family. Their flowers bloom early in the spring. Both plants are sweet and warming. They are helpful for sedating people who feel over-excited. The roots are rich in salicylates and have an action similar to that of aspirin.

The primrose stimulates and strengthens the lungs and helps clear them of mucus. It is helps in insomnia, stress, and migraines and other headaches. The Europeans who brought the tea to North America used it for nervous conditions. Add 5 to 10 drops of the essential oil to the bath at night to encourage sleep.

The cowslip is an attractive English wildflower with bright yellow, sweet-smelling, drooping blossoms. It is healing to the skin, helps sunburn, and fades freckles. The cooled tea can be used as a wash on problem skin. The flowers are helpful for nightmares, frenzies, nervousness, and trembling. Cowslip is a sedative, and the tea is used for pain (good for arthritis) and insomnia.

**Caution** Avoid ingesting the roots of primrose and cowslip if you are aspirin-sensitive. Do not use them if you are pregnant, taking blood-thinning medications, or have a history of epilepsy. Use the flowers, instead.

**Tea** Pour 1 cup (240 ml) of boiling water over 1 teaspoon (5 ml) of dried flowers or 2 teaspoons (10 ml) of fresh. Let steep for 5 minutes, strain, and sip. Drink up to 2 cups (480 ml) a day as needed.

## Valerian   (Valeriana officinalis)

Valerian is perhaps the best sedating nervine we have. Called nature's tranquilizer, it is used for hysteria, anxiety, headaches, nervous insomnia, palpitations, restlessness, and high blood pressure. It also improves concentration and helps elevate the mood while relaxing the body.

Sometimes called "all-heal", valerian is a traditional relaxant in pharmaceutical preparations and herbal teas. In China it has been used for colds. In the West it has been used to flavor tobacco, root beer, and liqueurs as well as to treat a variety of medical conditions stemming from nervous tension and migraines. The root is listed in the *British Herbal Pharmacoepia* as a sedative and an aid in nervous conditions.

A good night's sleep is imperative if the immune system is to remain strong. Valerian offers this without the possible hangover effects of a sleeping pill.

The herb is perennial, with a hollow, erect stem and short, thick, grayish, highly aromatic roots. It is strong, cooling, and bitter, and grows in damp meadows or mountainous regions.

**Caution** Take this tea no more than twice a day, or it may cause increased agitation. Taking it for more than 2 weeks without a break may lead to headaches and palpitations.

**Herbal Tea** Add ½ teaspoon (2.5 ml) of the powdered root to 2 cups (480 ml) of boiling water. Cover, and steep for 10 minutes. Add spices or honey, if desired. Stir, and sip slowly, leaving ½ inch (1.25 cm) at the bottom of the cup so that you don't ingest the sediment. Drink 1 to 2 cups (240–480 ml) a day as needed, no more.

## Wood Betony *(Stachys officinalis)*

Wood betony has intoxicating effects. The tea is cooling and bittersweet, good for body and soul, and has proved helpful in anxiety attacks, headaches, and other nervous disorders. It prevents bad dreams or nightmares and lowers blood pressure. It stimulates and cleanses the digestive system, purifies the blood, and is a natural painkiller.

Wood betony was used in the Middle Ages to ward off ill humors. It is native to the open woodlands and heaths of Scotland, and grows from Spain to the Caucasus. It is a hardy perennial with a musky odor, slightly bitter, but pleasant to drink. It blooms from July through August.

**Caution** An overdose of the tea can irritate the stomach. Do not take it if you are pregnant. Use the flower spikes and leaves.

**Tea** Use 1 teaspoon (5 ml) of dried leaves or 3 teaspoons (15 ml) of fresh. Cover with 1 cup (240 ml) of boiling water and steep for 5 to 6 minutes. It is slightly bitter, so you may want to add honey.

# Bach Flower Remedies

Dr. Edward Bach developed a blend of five different flower essences to be used during periods of severe stress or crisis. He called it "rescue remedy." You may take it by itself or in conjunction with an aromatherapy program. Place 3 drops of it under your tongue, or put the drops in ½ glass of water.

**Rockrose** fright or terror

**Clematis** withdrawal into fantasy or unclear thinking

**Impatiens** impatience, irritability, or impulsiveness

**Cherry Plum** loss of control, compulsiveness, or obsessiveness

**Star of Bethlehem** trauma of bad news, loss, or grief

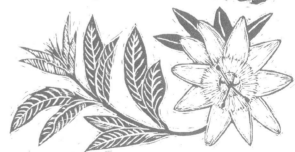

# Calming Essential Oils

## Aniseed  *(Pimpinella anisum)*

**Application**  Inhalation; sparingly in bath or massage oil

**Note**  Middle, balancing, spicy

**Caution**  Not for pregnant women, aniseed should be used cautiously by people with sensitive skin or high blood pressure. Overuse can cause irritation and dizziness.

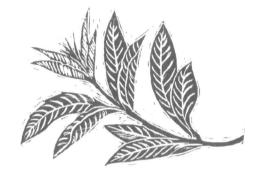

**Background**  Aniseed comes from an annual herb of the carrot family, with delicate leaves and flowers. It has a warm and spicy licoricelike aroma and taste. In Turkey, raki, a popular drink, is made from the seed. It is native to Greece and Egypt, widely cultivated in India and China, and popular in North America.

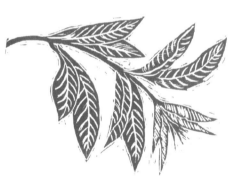

**Use**  A happy scent, it eases stress and worry, is good for hangovers and migraines, induces sweet dreams, and banishes nightmares. When both seeds and leaves are used, it is good for digestive problems like cramps and gas caused by nervous tension. Antiseptic, it flushes out impurities and is good for bronchial problems such as mucus and asthma. It is also good for stress-related nausea.

**Blend**  with lemon balm, neroli, and chamomile.

## Black Pepper  *(Piper nigrum)*

**Application**  Inhalation, massage

**Note**  Middle, balancing, spicy

**Caution**  Use it in moderation, or it can be irritating.

**Background**  Black pepper has been used for over 4,000 years both medicinally and in a culinary capacity. It is warming and healing for skin problems and respiratory and digestive complaints. In massage, it has been used for muscle aches and pains. It aids in reducing loss of appetite, nausea, and heartburn, and has been used to strengthen the body. Surprisingly, it is used in the perfume industry. The dried peppercorns come from a perennial woody vine native to tropical countries. It has a sharp, hot scent with a sweet undertone.

**Use**  It energizes the body, improves memory, and helps one cope with hard or difficult situations. It bestows calm courage and dispels nervous tension.

**Blend** with spice oils, cypress, and sandalwood.

## Calendula   (Calendula officinalis)

**Application**  Baths, herbal infusion, or compress

**Note**  Middle, balancing, herbaceous

**Background**  A favorite among herbalists, calendula is an annual with bright orange, daisylike flowers. It is a very powerful skin healer and has been used in high-class perfumery. It has an intense, sharp odor that's saffronlike and cooling. It is an erect, coarse, clammy plant that loves the sun and blooms from spring through fall. It is native to parts of Europe and North Africa eastward to Iran.

**Use**  This antiseptic essential oil is soothing to the skin and heals burns, cuts, and rashes, while it takes away pain. It comforts the heart and spirits and helps to calm weary or distressed persons who worry too much. It strengthens and helps bring on good dreams. It is good for headaches and red eyes. Use 5 to 10 drops of essential oil in the bath for anxiety or depression.

**Blend** with citrus and floral scents.

## Elemi   (Canarium luzonicum)

**Application**  Inhalation, compresses

**Note**  Base, grounding, resinous

**Background**  The poor man's frankincense, elemi is a resin exuded from a tropical tree. It has a faint lemon odor that is at once fresh and spicy. An oleoresin, it is used for skin care, in soaps and cosmetics, and as a fixative in perfumes. Sometimes it flavors food and alcoholic drinks. Medicinally, it helps relieve respiratory complaints. The ancient Egyptians used it to rejuvenate the skin, and it has been popular in Europe since the 1400s.

**Use**  A stimulant and tonic, it is good for nervous exhaustion and all stress-related conditions. In cool compresses it relaxes and rejuvenates facial skin and reduces wrinkles.

**Blend** with cinnamon, rosemary, and frankincense.

# Lemon Balm  *(Melissa officinalis)*

**Application**  Inhalation, compresses, herb in tea

**Note**  Middle, balancing, herbaceous

**Caution**  Do not use during pregnancy. Use low concentrations for sensitive skin. It is often adulterated, so check its purity.

**Background**  This sweet-scented herb grows to 2 feet (60 cm) and has bright green leaves and square stems. Native to the Mediterranean region, it is grown throughout the world. It is used extensively as a fragrance in beauty aids and as a flavoring for foods and drinks. The scent is lemony and refreshing.

**Use**  This herb soothes and calms mentally and physically. Similar to neroli or bergamot in its tonic properties, it aids in anxiety, stress, insomnia, tension, and shock. Slightly sedating, it is gentle and relaxing and a restorative for the nervous system. It refreshes, calms, and helps keep one from becoming depressed. Bitter and cooling, it is good for the lungs and for digestive problems, headaches, and dizziness. The herbalist John Gerard said that lemon balm "comforteth the heart," while other herbalists say it helps strengthen the memory and chases away all sadness. For a massage oil, add 5 to 10 drops to 2 teaspoons (10 ml) of almond oil. If you are having trouble with allergies, blend it with chamomile and inhale it.

**Blend** with chamomile, lavender, and geranium.

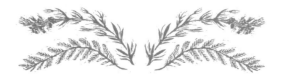

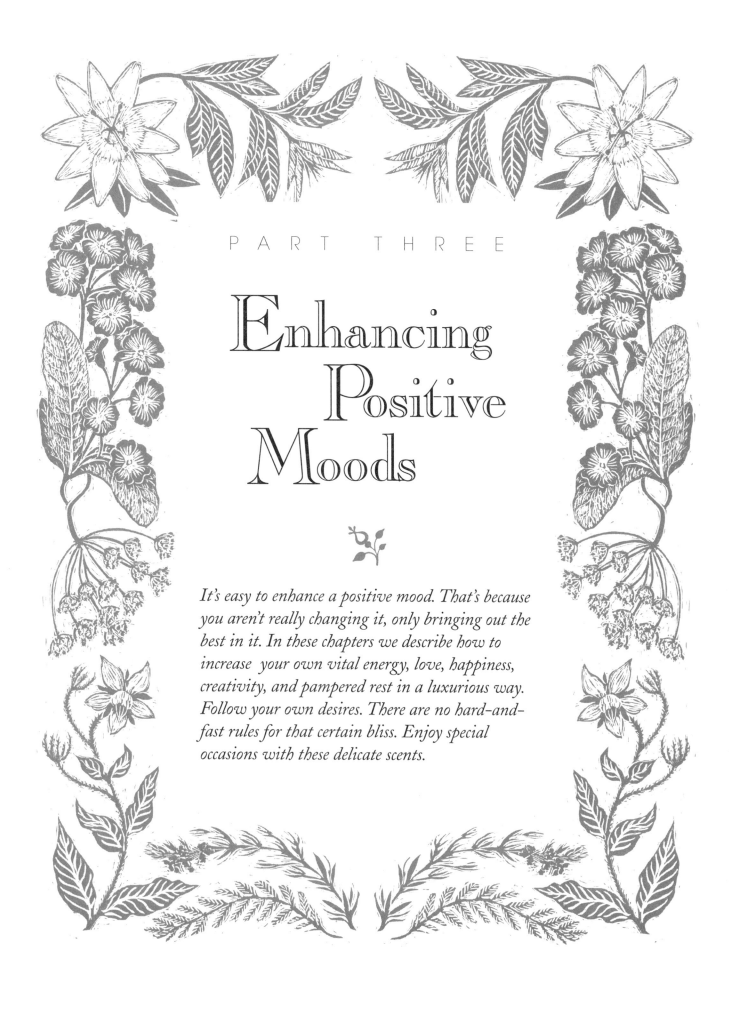

PART THREE

# Enhancing Positive Moods

*It's easy to enhance a positive mood. That's because you aren't really changing it, only bringing out the best in it. In these chapters we describe how to increase your own vital energy, love, happiness, creativity, and pampered rest in a luxurious way. Follow your own desires. There are no hard-and-fast rules for that certain bliss. Enjoy special occasions with these delicate scents.*

# CHAPTER EIGHT

# Getting Energized

*"Come, and trip it,*
*as ye go,*
*on the light*
*fantastic toe."*

—John Milton, "L'Allegro," 1631

Energy! Zest and zing! The vitality that makes us ready to tackle any challenge, to go and do and have fun. But some days we say, Where did it go?

If we weren't so worn out, we would finish building that play-fort for the kids, we would dance all night at that romantic little restaurant, we would do volunteer work, take classes, enrich our lives. Sometimes we are drained at the end of a tiring day. Sometimes we've had a hard week: hectic schedules, lack of sleep, poor nutrition, and emotional ups and downs. A balanced life has equal periods of work, rest, and recreation. When it gets out of balance, we have to stop and adjust it. For a quick start, we turn to the energizing essential oils.

## Fatigue

In this chapter we are not dealing with chronic fatigue. Chronic fatigue requires medical help. It is a condition of continual energy depletion caused by physical or mental problems, and its effects are far-reaching. A 1987 survey in the United States found that one out of every five women and one out of every six men complained of chronic fatigue. David S. Bell, M.D., lists six basic causes: stress and emotional upset, depression, medical illness, chronic-fatigue immune-dysfunction syndrome, sleep disorders, and poor nutrition. Possible physical causes include anemia, kidney problems, hidden thyroid dysfunction, and allergies. People who have chronic fatigue lasting more than a month should have a medical checkup. Fatigue is also one of the silent signals of high blood pressure.

What we are talking about in this chapter is simple everyday fatigue, the energy depletion that comes from the day-to-day routine. Fatigue is our body's way of telling us that we need to rest and recover. Our cells use energy to func-

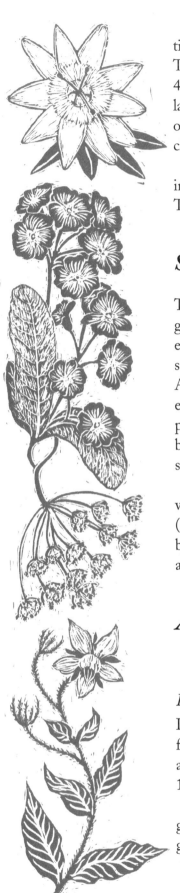

tion. They obtain this energy from the nutrients the body is fed. The cells that need the most energy are in the brain. That's why 4 hours of brain work can be more tiring than 8 hours of physical labor. Plenty of oxygen is needed, as energy is created only when oxygen burns the "fuel" (sugars) contained in nutrients. People with circulation problems often have reduced energy, too.

Energy begets energy. It puts oxygen into all parts of the body, including the brain. That's where stimulating essential oils come in. They get us moving, and that gets your energy rolling.

## Setting the Mood for Renewed Energy

The stimulating essential oils urge the body to take in more oxygen. Many of them have antiseptic and air-purifying qualities. They encourage deeper breathing and better blood circulation. They strengthen the body and immune system and make digestion easier. As helpful and useful as they are, these essential oils are very powerful and can be dangerous. The amounts administered and their period of use must be strictly limited. Only minimum doses should be given to the elderly, the ill, pregnant women, and children. Be sure to follow the guidelines for each oil listed in this chapter.

Time your therapy for early in the day or for a night when you want to stay up late. These essential oils will keep you awake (except lemon verbena, which helps you get a good night's sleep before an important day). Whenever your energy lags, choose an oil and a method that suit you.

## Application

### Inhalation

*Potpourri, Aroma Lamp, Steam & Scented Paper*
If you want to get up refreshed and ready to go, try an electric diffuser with a timer. Set it to start shortly before you awake. You can also light a simmering potpourri burner (filled with water and 5 to 10 drops of essential oil) to scent the air as you breakfast and dress.

If you come home at the end of the day exhausted, one way to get an energy boost is to keep an aroma lamp or potpourri burner going for about an hour. Another is to use steam inhalation. Pour hot water into a bowl, add 3 to 5 drops of essential oil, then cover your head and the bowl with a towel. Close your eyes and inhale deeply for 2 to 5 minutes, no longer. You will immediately feel energized and uplifted.

To get a boost during the day, if you work with books or papers, put several drops onto a paper bookmark, enclose this in plastic overnight to let the scent infuse the paper, and keep it with you for whenever you need extra zing. Personal stationery can be infused in the same way. If you are on the go or on your feet all day, you can purchase aromatherapy jewelry to infuse with scent and wear during the day; or simply add 1 or 2 drops of essential oil (only pure nonresinous oils, or they may stain your clothes) to your sleeve or lapel.

## Absorption

**Caution** Two of the essential oils listed here should not be used on the skin: cinnamon bark and ginger. The rest can be used in stimulating baths, in moderation, 5 to 10 drops or as specified. These baths should be taken no more than once a week, for no longer than 30 minutes. Overdosing can overload the body and increase stress levels.

### Massage Oils

Massage oils can also be made, as long as the caution statements for each essential oil are observed. Peppermint and thyme are both good in massage oils. Use 10 drops in 2 fluid ounces (60 ml) of a carrier oil such as sweet almond or olive. Peppermint is antispasmodic, good for sore muscles, and helpful in draining the lymphatics. Thyme is very good for arthritis and weakness.

## Ingestion

### Herbal Teas & Tinctures

Peppermint and thyme make good teas. Peppermint is refreshing and energizing and stimulates the appetite. Herbalists say that thyme helps the digestion and supports the formation of white blood cells, so stimulating the immune system. Use 1 teaspoon (5 ml) of dried or 3 teaspoons (15 ml) of fresh herbs (use both leaves and flowers of peppermint) to 1 cup (240 ml) of boiling water. Steep for 5 minutes.

Use the following three aromatic herbs in a tincture to electrify your body back into action. You may not want to take them after 3 P.M., as they can keep you up way into the night.

### Cayenne  (Capsicum frutescens)

This is a very hot herb. Originally from India, it arrived in North America from Central and South America and was popular in the 19th century for its warming properties. It is a spice from the pepper family that is now grown in gardens the world over and is used to make Tabasco and other sauces.

High in vitamins C and A, this oddly pointed fruit is a stimulating nerve tonic and promotes sweating. Two doses of the tincture in warm water can banish a cold. It is a digestive and appetite stimulant, it relieves indigestion, and it eases the pain of shingles, arthritis, and migraines.

**Caution** Avoid this if you have intestinal disorders, like ulcers or bowel disease.

**Tincture** Add ¼ ounce (7 g) to 10 fluid ounces (300 ml) of apple cider vinegar. For a stimulant or to quiet nausea, add 5 to 10 drops to ½ cup (120 ml) of warm water. Drink this no more than twice a day.

### Ginger  (Zingiber officinale)

**Tincture** Slice the root thinly and cover it with vodka. Place it in a sunny window for 3 to 4 weeks. Strain. Take 2 to 10 drops as needed for loss of energy, indigestion, or nausea.

# Energizing Essential Oils

## Cinnamon  (Cinnamomum zeylanicum)

**Application** Inhalation with a diffuser or steam vaporizer

**Note** Base, nourishing, spicy

**Caution** The essential oil obtained from the bark is very powerful and should not be used on the skin or given to pregnant women. The elderly or very weak should use it in moderation.

**Background** The tree is native to Sri Lanka and Madagascar. Related to the laurel, it is a tropical evergreen with thick bark and shiny green leaves that have a spicy smell when rubbed. The essential oil made from the leaves is much milder than that from the bark and can be used in skin preparations. We use the essential oil of the bark for inhalation.

Cinnamon is used in fragrances and as a flavor in many things, including Coca-Cola and dental preparations. For centuries the Chinese have used it in a decoction for weakened energy. The inner bark is scraped off, made into little rolls or sticks, and dried. It used to be a rare and expensive spice. The ancient Greeks made a drink called hippocras of cinnamon and other spices mixed with sugared wine. It was said to be a most invigorating tonic.

**Use** Cinnamon is comforting, warming and strengthening to the body and mind, and energizing. It helps dispel feelings of isolation and tension. Its warm, spicy, sweet scent is pungent and potent. It aids in reducing exhaustion, sluggish digestion, circulation, debility, and anorexia. It is a room purifier. Be careful to follow the precautions given here and to use the amounts recommended under Inhalation (pp. 83–84).

**Blend** with ylang-ylang, coriander, and citrus oils.

## Citronella    *(Cymbopogon nardus)*

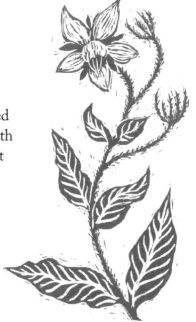

**Application** Inhalation, in a vaporizer

**Note** Top, fresh, herbaceous

**Caution** Do not use it during pregnancy or on sensitive skin.

**Background** Citronella comes from a tall, aromatic, perennial grass native to Sri Lanka and now cultivated widely. It has a fresh, powerful, lemony scent. In North America it is known mainly as an ingredient in insect repellent, but in many cultures it is a stimulant and a cooling agent for fevers. Chinese medicine uses it for rheumatic pain.

**Use** It has a clear, uplifting quality and is good for nervous exhaustion, simple physical fatigue, headaches, and pain, but should be used sparingly. It purifies the room.

**Blend** with geranium, lemon, and bergamot.

## Copaiba Balsam    *(Copaifera officinalis)*

**Application** Inhalation, perfumes

**Note** Base, nourishing, resinous

**Background** Copaiba resin (not a true balsam) is collected from holes drilled in the tree trunk. The oil and resin are produced in Brazil and Colombia. The essential oil has a sweet, balsamic, yet peppery odor, but the crude resin, which we are using, is woody and spicy. It is one of the most plentiful of perfume ingredients.

**Use** This stimulant is an energizer and dispels exhaustion and other stress-related problems. It also purifies the room.
**Blend** with ylang-ylang, vanilla, and jasmine.

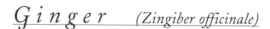

## $G\ i\ n\ g\ e\ r$   *(Zingiber officinale)*

**Application** Inhalation, in a diffuser; sparingly ingested as a digestive
**Note** Base, nourishing, spicy
**Caution** Ginger is not recommended in skin preparations. It can be used for morning sickness, but sparingly: only 1 drop in ½ cup (120 ml) of warm water to energize, dispel nausea, and calm stomach problems.
**Background** Originally from tropical Asia, ginger is an erect perennial with tuberous roots that was introduced into the West by the Spaniards. The spicy root is used. For centuries considered a medicinal, it is still used to modify the action of any herbal remedy. It is listed as a digestive in the *British Herbal Pharmacopoeia*. The oleoresin is used in cosmetics and perfumery. The root is sometimes candied.
**Use** Ginger is regarded by Chinese herbalists as high in yang energy. Less harsh than black pepper, it sharpens the senses and is a stimulating tonic. It is a restorative, good for physical and nervous exhaustion, nausea, and low blood circulation. It warms, aids in loss of appetite, and acts as a mild painkiller. It purifies the room.
**Blend** with rosewood, orange, and other citrus oils.

## $L\ e\ m\ o\ n\ \ V\ e\ r\ b\ e\ n\ a$   *(Lippia citriodora)*

**Application** Inhalation, in a diffuser or aroma lamp; herb in tea
**Note** Middle, flowing, herbaceous
**Caution** Avoid it in pregnancy. It can cause sun sensitivity. Lemon verbena is often adulterated, so check its purity.
**Background** This tender perennial is a fragile-looking little bush with light green leaves and tiny white blossoms. Very sensitive to the cold, it is often grown as a houseplant. In France it is a popular tea. The oil is often used in colognes, perfumes, and bath products.
**Use** Lemon verbena is calming, soothing, and refreshing, best used at the end of the day. It relieves stress, renews energy, and quickly overcomes tiredness, disinterest, and apathy. Especially good for women, it helps generate enthusiasm, strengthens the heart, and aids in reducing digestive weakness, nausea, and dizziness. A tonic but not a stimulant, it induces restful sleep, so that you

wake up renewed the next day. It is also an air purifier.

**Blend** with neroli, hyssop, and myrtle.

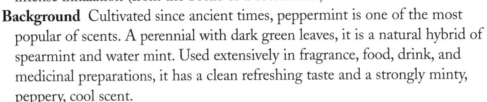

## *Peppermint*  *(Mentha piperita)*

**Application**  Inhalation

**Note**  Top, fresh, herbaceous

**Caution**  Do not give peppermint to pregnant women or children under age 2. Do not administer it for more than 1 week at a time, or it may cause nervous disorders. Use it sparingly in skin preparations. Avoid inhaling it for prolonged periods, limiting its use to 1 hour in room diffusers or 5 minutes of intense inhalation (from the bottle or a cotton ball).

**Background**  Cultivated since ancient times, peppermint is one of the most popular of scents. A perennial with dark green leaves, it is a natural hybrid of spearmint and water mint. Used extensively in fragrance, food, drink, and medicinal preparations, it has a clean refreshing taste and a strongly minty, peppery, cool scent.

**Use**  Peppermint is considered a great mental stimulant, rousing the senses, clearing the head, and enhancing self-confidence. It is penetrating and calming. It stimulates the circulation, the nervous system, and the draining of the lymphatic system. A good digestive and pain reliever, it is efficacious against headaches, fever, dizziness, vomiting or nausea, and motion sickness. In massage, it helps cramping muscles (see Absorption, p. 84). It purifies the room. To use it as an energizer, add 3 drops to the bath early in the day.

**Blend**  with lavender, black pepper, and rosemary.

## *Rosemary*  *(Rosmarinus officinalis)*

**Application**  Inhalation, in a diffuser; absorption, in massage oils

**Note**  Middle, flowing, herbaceous

**Caution**  Avoid use when pregnant or if you have high blood pressure or epilepsy.

**Background**  The stems, leaves, and flowers are used. A native to the Mediterranean, now grown in California, Russia, the Middle East, Britain, France, Spain, and China, rosemary is a shrubby evergreen plant, a tender perennial with needle-shaped leaves. It has a strong camphorous odor. It is used extensively as a scent in soaps and cosmetics, as an antiseptic in cleaning supplies, and as a flavoring for foods and drinks.

**Use** Rosemary is strengthening, centering, and invigorating. It is deemed a restorative, good for exhaustion, weakness, muscular pains (as from overwork or arthritis), headaches, fainting, and mental fatigue. It is listed in the *British Herbal Pharmacopoeia* as good for depressive states with weakness and general debility. It improves memory ("rosemary is for remembrance"). It is also good for chest congestion. A general tonic, it stimulates blood circulation, increases blood pressure, strengthens the heart and nervous system, and helps prevent mood swings. It is a support in stressful times, since it is uplifting and energizing and leads to euphoria. Rosemary dispels sluggishness and clears the head. It centers one during meditation. To use it as an energizer, add 10 drops to the bath. It also purifies the air.

**Blend** with basil, peppermint, and lemon.

## *Thyme* *(Thymus zygis or Thymus vulgaris)*

**Application** Inhalation, bath, massage
**Note** Top, fresh, herbaceous
**Caution** Avoid thyme in pregnancy. Use it in moderation, particularly on sensitive skin.
**Background** Thyme is one of the oldest medicinal plants in the Western herbal repertoire. An evergreen perennial native to Spain and the Mediterranean, it is found throughout the world in many different scented varieties. Thyme has proven disinfectant qualities and is used in mouthwashes, gargles, toothpastes, fragrance, and food and drink.
**Use** Thyme supplies energy in times of physical or mental weakness. It reduces tiredness and builds strength after illness. Herbalists say it calms the nerves. Inhaled, it aids concentration. It is revitalizing when you feel nervous debility, stress-related fatigue, and exhaustion. It bestows courage, clarity, and sharpness. Thyme also helps mild depression, headaches, indigestion, and respiratory problems (it is a good decongestant). It has a pungent, slightly bitter taste and a strongly medicinal scent.

Thyme is good in massage (see Absorption). Use 3 drops in the bath to ease arthritic pain and to gain energy and strength.
**Blend** with lemon balm, rosemary, and citrus oils.

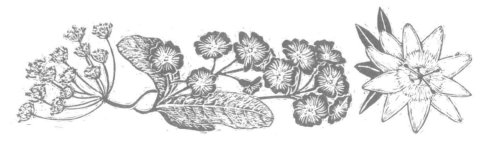

# CHAPTER NINE

# Love, Sex & Aphrodisiacs

*"A heart as soft,*
*a heart as kind,*
*a heart as sound and free*
*as in the whole world*
*thou canst find,*
*that heart I'll give to thee."*

—Robert Herrick, "To Anthea Who May
Command Him Anything," 1648

We can't predict where or when love will strike, but strike it will. As country music tells us, love, true love, is painful. All too often the object of our desire does not reciprocate. And in the real world, even partners who have long been together find that romantic feelings can wax and wane. That's why people, since ancient times, have tried spells, lures, potions, elixirs—anything within the power of imagination—to attract or bind the object of their desire to them. We see such Puckish magic afoot in Shakespeare's *A Midsummer Night's Dream.* Love attachments seem sudden and ridiculous. A woman falls in love with the donkey-ears of a fool. Two youths spin away from their mad love of one girl to become clingingly enamored with her best friend, a girl they once disdained.

## Ah, Love!

*Aphrodisiacs* are named after Aphrodite, the Greek goddess of love. She held sway over all human matters involving love and lust. To the Greek and Roman poets, she was the all-powerful force that shaped men's lives. Folklore has many tales of aphrodisiacs. Some have been very strange concoctions, containing, for example, crocodile semen or decaying matter from corpses. Others are more appealing, and most of these involve scent.

Perfuming to attract the opposite sex is an ancient art. The Egyptians created elaborate rituals of love that included bathing, veils, perfumes, cosmetics, and

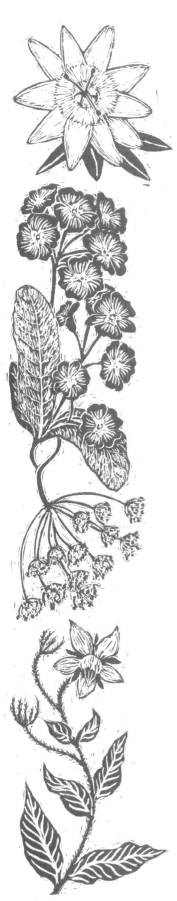

costly jewelry. One famous user of scent was Cleopatra, who enticed her beloved Marc Antony with exotic odors. The Romans applied perfume lavishly. They didn't merely dab it on pulse points. They perfumed their heads, hair, garments, and even the air, and ate spices to sweeten their breath. Street vendors peddled love potions containing hot spices and herbs steeped in wines. In Arabia, erotic manuals stressed the importance of perfumes for both men and women.

In ancient Egypt, 18th century Europe, and in parts of the Orient to this day, some women have followed a practice of inserting small perfumed pads inside themselves before intercourse, to arouse and excite their lovers and enhance the sexual experience. (We do not recommend anyone try this, in view of the danger of damaging delicate tissues, causing an allergic reaction, or even toxic shock.) In a part of Australia, the aboriginal men place the crushed root of a particular tree (*Pittosporum venuloseum*) outside the women's huts. These roots are powerfully aromatic, and the scent is believed to arouse sexual excitement.

## Pheromones

Western science hasn't put much faith in the existence of truly aphrodisiac properties, but it is beginning to learn things about the biological significance of scent. The secretion of *pheromones* has been discovered in insects and in higher forms of life as well. Pheromones are chemicals that communicate signals, one of the signals being readiness to mate. The term was coined by Adolf Butenandt and his co-workers in 1959 to describe the sex-stimulating chemical signals secreted by the female silk moth.

We humans, too, have our signals. One of our skin glands, the *apocrine*, is being investigated as the source of smells that may affect human interactions. These glands appear on our hands, cheeks, scalp, breast areolas, and wherever there is body hair. And these scent glands are functional only after puberty, when the time has come for us to begin our search for mates. They secrete actively during times of nervousness or excitement. The nose, when stimulated by these pheromones, affects the portion of the brain called the *hypothalamus*. This in turn stimulates the body to respond with sexual feelings and mood.

There are also gender differences, with a purpose. Men's apocrine glands are larger than women's, but women have a keener sense of smell, especially during ovulation. This tells us that at the time that they are most likely to conceive, women have a sharp sense of smell, while men are really pumping the smells out for the purpose of attracting them.

### Sex & the Odor-Confused

Researchers at the University of Bern, Switzerland, have discovered that scent attraction has another interesting aspect. Women seem to be the most attracted to the scents of males whose immune systems are most different from their own. The researchers conclude that children born from parents with such varied biological factors would have strong immune systems—a way of strengthening the species. And if you have wondered why there seems to be so much divorce today, we may have a reason. The study further found that women on birth control pills seemed to become "odor-confused" and react in the opposite way, being attracted to men with similar immune systems. What happens, then, when the woman goes off the Pill? Does she wake up one day with a mate whose scent no longer attracts her?

### Plant Mimics

And what about the scents we get from plants? Aromatherapists assert that some essential oils contain volatile substances that mimic the human sex pheromones. So if we know which plant chemicals affect human sexual moods, we can use them to our advantage next time we pine for love.

## Setting the Mood for Love

Eros, the son of Aphrodite, was called Cupid by the Romans, who claimed that he shot his arrows at hapless humans to make them fall in love. Supposedly he couldn't hit those who were always in a rush, restless, or fidgety. But if he happened upon someone who was still and fully relaxed, then he could strike with ease. As the Emperor Nero once said, love is a mental condition fostered by leisure.

In setting the mood for romance, then, we must create an atmosphere of relaxation. A few luxurious touches help, too: a cozy table for two set with your best, appealing food, some wine if you like it, soft music, and plenty of scent filling the air. The traditional aphrodisiac oils come mostly from tropical flowers or herbs with a warming, relaxing, yet stimulating quality. You may add essential oils to an aromatherapy lamp, or set out potpourri, scented candles, or fresh flowers. Later in the evening, you might use a massage oil, prepare a warm sensual bath for two, or toss rose petals across the bed.

92

Make sure that you choose ways of savoring each other's company. Romance is successful when you think of the other person's needs. Setting the mood doesn't start in the evening but begins days ahead of time. Anticipate your night of love. Send out your own signals—hugs, touches, kisses, compliments, little gifts. Then let the evening unfold in a deliciously scented cloud. Your night of romance will be a passionate success—soon followed by more.

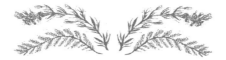

# Application

## Inhalation & Absorption

### Scented Candles, Potpourri & More

Scented candles, with their soft and mysterious light, immediately create a mood. For a delicate scented touch, you might place a few drops of essential oil on the bedsheets or put around small bowls of potpourri. Scent burners, aroma lamps, and diffusers also effectively perfume a room. Just don't overdo. Too much scent can be a turn-off. You don't want to overwhelm your object of love.

Discreetly use some perfume or cologne on yourself. This is good both for attracting a new interest and renewing a long-term relationship. Perfumes and colognes are not hard to make, but it takes time to create the perfect blend. Women's perfumes and men's colognes differ merely in their essential oils and their strength. Women will want to wear the more floral scents, in heavier concentrations. Men will probably choose woody, herbaceous, or spicy blends. Colognes use herbal waters, so they are lighter than perfumes.

### "Aphrodisiac" Perfume

Use either a single essential oil or a blend. Have ready a glass perfume bottle or a spray atomizer. To 1 fluid ounce (30 ml) of vodka add 100 drops of essential oil. Next add 20 drops of cold-pressed castor oil as a fixative (this also blends well with the alcohol). Seal. Let it stand for 2 weeks before using it.

### Cologne or Aftershave

Put 2 fluid ounces (60 ml) of vodka and 50 drops of essential oil into a nice-looking glass jar. Make a strong herbal or spice water: to ¼ cup (60 ml) of boiling water add 1 teaspoon (5 ml) of a dried aromatic herb of your choice or ½ teaspoon (2.5 ml) of spice or 1 cinnamon stick. Steep for 5 to 6 minutes. Strain. Add it to the vodka and essential oils. Add 20 to 30 drops of cold-pressed castor oil, and blend well. Splash it on freely after shaving.

## Romantic Baths

Choose from sexy baths–perhaps for two–and enjoyable aromatic massages. Romance, of course, depends on aromas compatible with both of you. So heed personal preferences and any allergies!

A sexy soak in aromatic bathwater is by far the most enjoyable way to get into a romantic mood. The scent is not only inhaled but absorbed, and the warm water creates a relaxed and receptive state while increasing blood circulation. You can also use a Jacuzzi if you want to include a partner. Here's a great way to disperse the scent throughout the water. Mix 6 to 12 drops of essential oil or oils with 1 teaspoon (5 ml) of mild shampoo (for a bubble bath) or 1 teaspoon (5 ml) of jojoba oil. Add it as the tub fills, and swirl it around.

**Caution** Do not exceed 6 to 12 drops total of essential oil in a bath.

## Romantic Massage Oils

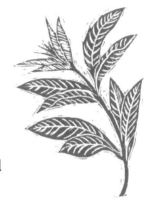

Massage is a wonderful loving touch. We all need that. Premature babies in incubators have been found to gain weight faster when nurses touch and stroke them daily. And when touch is used between lovers, it deepens their loving mood. You don't have to be an expert. With your fingertips, rub scented oil into your lover's skin; then let your lover do the same for you, while you both absorb and inhale the heavenly aromas.

To make the massage as enjoyable as possible, see that the room is warm, without drafts, and dimly lit. Have towels and robes handy (you may want to place towels over the bed linens so that the oils don't stain them). Before applying the oil, pour it into your hand to warm it—cold chills can nix romance.

If you want to go deeply into the art of massage, there are many books and videos on the subject.

### Massage Oil Recipe

To make your own massage oil, add 15 to 20 drops of essential oil or oils to 1 fluid ounce (30 ml) of any vegetable oil. Add 1 to 2 vitamin E capsules (take a pin and prick the capsule, then squeeze the vitamin E into the mix; or simply use bottled vitamin E). Blend well.

## Ingestion

### Herbal Tinctures

Sexual vitality can sometimes be a problem, especially for men. If a man has trouble achieving or maintaining an erection, it is of course hard to maintain the mood of romance. About 80 percent of impotence in men comes from mental or emotional factors or from transitory problems like stress, alcohol, blood-pressure medications, and plain fatigue. Age shouldn't cause problems, although normally a male slows down after age 50. But older men can be just as vital and have just as satisfying a love life as always, even into advanced age. A man should make sure he doesn't have physical problems such as diabetes, or prostate or cardiovascular disease. If he is merely in need of a little boost in the area of love, he may try the following aphrodisiac herbs in tincture form. These three herbs help impotence and act as circulatory stimulants as well as hormonal balancers.

### Damiana   (Turnera diffusa)

Use the leaves of this herb, which is believed to strengthen the nervous system and is very good for increasing sensitivity to touch. It has long been used as an aphrodisiac, a tonic to the central nervous system, and a hormone balancer. It aids in reducing impotence and sexual dysfunction due to depression. Since it can interfere with iron absorption, be careful if you are anemic.

**Tincture**   Place ¼ ounce (7 g) of dried leaf in 10 fluid ounces (300 ml) of vodka. Let it steep for 2 weeks. Strain. Take 1 to 2 eyedroppersful (1–2 ml) in a glass of water two to three times per day.

### Ginseng   (Panax ginseng)

The root from the Asian ginseng helps to stimulate production of the male sex hormone testosterone. (The somewhat less strong American ginseng *Panax quinquefolius* can be used if the Asian kind is hard to obtain.) It also invigorates and bestows vitality and energy. It is best for someone who is merely stressed or exhausted and wants to get some sexual energy back quickly.

**Tincture**   Add 1 ounce (28 g) of powdered root to 10 fluid ounces (300 ml) of vodka. Let it steep for 3 weeks. Strain. Take 1 teaspoonful (5 ml) up to three times per day. Ginseng can be taken on a long-term basis.

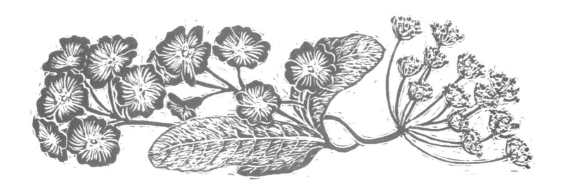

# Loverly Essential Oils

## Clary Sage (Salvia sclarea)

**Application** Inhalation

**Note** Top, fresh, herbaceous

**Caution** Some people find this quite intoxicating. Overdosing will cause headaches. Don't drive or operate machinery after using it. Don't mix it with alcohol, and don't use it if you are pregnant.

**Background** A stout biennial with hairy leaves and small blue flowers, clary sage is native to southern Europe and is cultivated worldwide. It has been used in perfumery and in the production of wines with muscatel flavor. It has a sweet scent, musty and almost smoky. In earlier times the seeds were ground and added to wine for the purpose of inciting lust.

**Use** A warming, soothing essential oil, it creates euphoria in some and deep relaxation in others. It helps in cases of sexual problems, opening the mind and getting rid of tension and headaches. It is stimulating and revitalizing, yet induces tranquility. It slows the brain and has been regarded as helpful for both impotence and frigidity, although it is used more for female sexual dysfunction, especially for women apprehensive of sexual encounters. It is also good for elderly lovers or for those suffering mid-life sexual crises.

**Blend** with bergamot and jasmine.

## Cumin (Cuminum cyminum)

**Application** Sensual baths, massage oils

**Note** Middle, flowing, spicy

**Caution** Don't use it during pregnancy. Since it causes sun sensitivity, don't expose the skin to sun after treatment.

**Background** The dried fruits or seeds of this delicate annual are used to make the essential oil. The plant has slender stems, feathery leaves, and oblong seeds that are a traditional Middle Eastern spice and an ingredient in curry.

It is closely related to coriander. Cumin was used as a stimulant in ayurvedic medicine. Native to Egypt, it is much used in Mexican cooking and is a seasoning for food and drink. Its scent is spicy, musky, and warming, and it is a secret ingredient in perfumes that are said to inspire lust.

**Use** The scent of cumin is a very powerful aphrodisiac, inciting romantic notions and bestowing energy. It stimulates the circulation, acts as a nervine and tonic, and banishes migraines and other headaches.

**Blend** with lavender, galbanum, and rosewood.

# Gardenia  (*Gardenia* species)

**Application**  Inhalation

**Note**  Middle, flowing, floral

**Caution**  This essential oil can be difficult to obtain commercially. You might think of growing your own gardenia.

**Background**  Used in high-class perfumery, gardenia is a decorative, tender, perennial bush grown for ornamental purposes. Its fragrant white flowers are sometimes used in corsages. It is evergreen, with dark green leathery leaves. It can be a successful houseplant if kept moist and warm.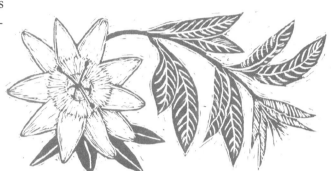
It belongs to the madder family and demands a high-acid soil. It is native to the Far East, India, and China. The Chinese prize it as a warming tea, but efforts at commercial production have failed so far. The flowers have a rich, sweet floral scent, reminiscent of jasmine.

**Use**  Highly aphrodisiac, gardenia enhances romantic longing. If you grow your own bush, pick the gardenia buds before they flower and dry them in a darkened room out of the sun. They have a sweet strawberry scent.

**Essential Oil**  Pack a jar with the dried buds, cover them with good vodka, and shake the jar daily for 3 weeks. Strain. Place the strained vodka in the freezer for several hours. The essential oil of the gardenia should have floated to the top. Skim this off with a spoon and store it in a small dark bottle.

**Blend**  with ylang-ylang, rose, and any spice oil.

# Jasmine  (*Jasminum officinale*)

**Application**  Perfume, massage

**Note**  Base, nourishing, floral

**Caution**  Pregnant women should not use it. Also, it can attract more attention than desired from the opposite sex.

**Background**  This evergreen vine with delicate bright green leaves and star-shaped, very fragrant flowers has been called "queen of the night" in India. Rightly so, for the fragrance calls to mind mystery and majesty. The dried flowers have been used in teas, and the oil in food products, drinks, and extensively in high-class perfumery and cosmetics. Jasmine was imported to

Europe from Persia in the 16th century. Its scent is intensely rich, warm, and floral.

**Use** The essential oil of jasmine is very expensive, but powerful. A little goes a long way. In fact, the more gentle the scent, the more effective. It increases the attractiveness of the wearer. Very aphrodisiac, erotic, and sensual, it is capable of immediately changing one's mood and opening one up to new love and total abandon. A confidence booster, it is good for someone with low self-esteem, bestowing euphoria, confidence, and optimism. It is relaxing and sedating and is an antidepressant. It aids in postnatal sadness and in getting back to normal sexual activity.

**Blend** with all oils, especially ylang-ylang and rose.

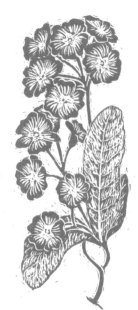

## *Patchouli* *(Pogostemon cablin)*

**Application** Bath oils, body lotions, perfumes
**Note** Base, nourishing, herbaceous
**Background** Native to tropical Asia, patchouli is a perennial bushy herb with hairy stems, large fragrant leaves, and white flowers. It has been used in the East to scent linens, and medicinally in China, Japan, and Malaysia for headaches and nausea. It is an ingredient in cosmetics. Patchouli has a strong sensual odor, deep, rich, and musty, that is sometimes used as a masking agent for unpleasant tastes or smells.
**Blend** with basil, pine, and rose.

## *Rockrose* *(Cistus ladanifer)*

**Application** Inhalation, massage
**Note** Base, nourishing, woody
**Caution** Avoid using it in pregnancy.
**Background** This bush has rough dark green leaves with delicate flowers. The twigs and stems are used to make the essential oil. Originally from the Mediterranean, rockrose resembles the wild rose but is unrelated to it. Its scent is warm, deep, and spicy, yet woody.
**Use** This erotic scent is soothing to the soul. It helps break the ice in new relationships and rekindle warmth when one partner has turned cold and emotionally distant. It also aids in frigidity, and it is good for the skin.
**Blend** with ylang-ylang and any spicy oil.

# Rosewood  *(Aniba rosaeodora)*

**Application** Inhalation, perfume

**Note** Base, nourishing, woody

**Background** This medium-size tropical evergreen with reddish bark and yellow flowers is native to the Amazon and tropical rain forests. Formerly the French used it for woodworking. Today most of the wood goes to Japan to be made into chopsticks. It has a sweet, woody fragrance and is used extensively in perfumery.

**Use** Very balancing when inhaled, this is a good substitute for the more expensive rose essential oil, although less powerful. Rosewood is comforting, abates mood swings, and aids in lessening feelings of neglect and abandonment. It helps relieve sadness and inspires love. An aphrodisiac that energizes the autonomic nervous system, it is tonic and combats stress and frigidity. It is also good for the skin.

**Blend** with most oils.


# Ylang-Ylang  *(Cananga odorata)*

### (Also called ILANG-ILANG)

**Application** Baths, massage, perfumes

**Note** Base, nourishing, floral

**Caution** Use it sparingly, since overuse causes headaches and nausea.

**Background** Flowers from this tall evergreen are very sweet-smelling and floral, yet soft and spicy, and are used extensively in perfume. Some people find the oil too sweet and prefer to blend it with other oils. In Malayan its name means "flower of flowers." In Indonesia the beds of newlyweds traditionally are covered with this bloom. The flowers are less fragrant in the wild, and the tree is extensively cultivated to produce large yellowish white blooms.

**Use** Ylang-ylang has a very erotic, very feminine scent. It induces euphoria and reduces anxiety. It is strengthening and calming, a sedative for the nerves and a stimulant for the circulation. A nervine that soothes frustration and anger, it balances hormones, and warms those who are emotionally cold. It can help men get in touch with their emotions and softer side.

**Blend** with most oils, especially orange.

# CHAPTER TEN

# Relaxation & Restful Sleep

*"And flights of angels sing thee to thy rest!"*

—William Shakespeare,
*Hamlet*, 1600

There is nothing better than a long and refreshing sleep that lets you wake up full of energy and greet the new day with joy. Sometimes, however, a good night's sleep seems ever so elusive. You just can't unwind. The day's events whirl through your mind, and you worry over the day to come. The longer the night grows, the wider awake you become. You are suffering from that pesty, irritating complaint, insomnia.

Let's make it clear that the recommendations in this chapter are not for severe sleep disorders, the so-called short-term insomnia caused by psychological stress that can last several weeks or the chronic insomnia that lasts months or years. These extreme forms of insomnia require professional advice. Organizations worlwide can refer you to a specialist. In the United States, the American Sleep Disorders Association in Rochester, Minnesota, and the National Sleep Foundation in Los Angeles, California, may be helpful.

## Wide Awake

If you're not sure that you have severe insomnia, try the remedies here, making sure to observe the cautions. Keep in mind that pregnancy and menopause can cause changes in sleep patterns, as can any medications you are taking. If you think your insomnia is caused by a particular kind of stress, you may want to choose some of the essential oils recommended for that stress and blend them with some of those suggested in this chapter. If you are still experiencing sleep problems after 3 weeks, you should seek a physician's advice.

### Transient Insomnia

Essential oils can be very effective in transient insomnia. This annoying condition may be brought on by minor stresses like bad sleeping habits, overindul-

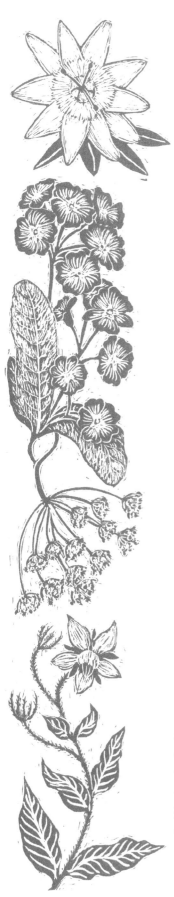

gence in food or drink, interrupted sleep, overwork, an unsympathetic spouse, minor illness, worries, and the demands of child-rearing. Generally it lasts no more than a few nights—perhaps recurring over a period of weeks—if left to run its course. But we can prevent the hassle of those sleepless nights by using the essential oils.

Most of us have gone through such times. Researchers estimate that over half the population of the United States suffers intermittent sleep disturbances. Women may be especially affected, according to a report by the (U.S.) National Center on Sleep Disorders Research. It cites hormonal fluctuations related to the menstrual cycle and menopause, along with pregnancy-related changes. Surveys show that over 40 percent of women over 40 years old confront insomnia or restless nights from time to time.

An impending attack of mild insomnia gives no warning signs. One night you find that the clock reads 2:30 A.M., and you still haven't drifted off to dreamland. You toss and turn, and look at your sleeping spouse with resentment. You wearily punch your pillow and try to "will" yourself to sleep, only to feel more and more frustrated and angry as you lie there in an agony of wakefulness. You're tired, right? You have things to do the next day, right? Why can't you go to sleep? Or perhaps you have a child who is restless and can't seem to get into a good sleep routine. This interrupts your own sleep schedule. You worry about your child's sleeplessness and wonder if the next day the child will be cranky and irritable, and if you will be, too.

## Dangers of Insomnia

Sleep researchers say that concern is valid, for even one night of fitful sleep can make us grumpy and unable to concentrate well, affecting our performance at work or school. The elderly may find that mild depression, life-style changes, certain chronic health conditions, and perhaps lack of proper activity and exercise lead to a mild insomnia that affects their moods and thereby their social relationships and quality of life. Lack of proper sleep can even be dangerous. Over 100,000 car accidents a year are caused by drivers who fall asleep or become drowsy. And studies show that shift workers, who may chronically not get enough restful sleep, have an increased risk of infertility, heart disease, and digestive or gastrointestinal disorders.

Only we ourselves know how much sleep we need to feel good

the next day. The average adult needs 8 to 9 hours a night, but most get only 7 hours and many get 6 hours or less. Newborn babies need 17 to 18 hours per day, while older children do best on 9 to 10 hours. Dr. Stanley Coren, a neuropsychologist at the University of British Columbia, estimates that we accumulate a sleep debt of about 500 hours a year, due in part to our clock-driven life.

After a rocky night, sometimes we turn to sleep medications. Over 10 million people in the United States alone obtain prescriptions for sleep aids. Yet these sleeping pills don't work very well. They make us groggy the next day, and we don't really feel refreshed when we wake up. Studies show that these medications may make matters worse, either by interfering with the brain's sleep cycles, by increasing the severity of the insomnia, or by starting up a cycle of addiction to the medication. Sleep medications interfere with the phases of sleep. One of those phases is the deep stage of REM (rapid eye movement), which is associated with dreaming. According to sleep researchers, this is an important restorative stage, physically as well as mentally and spiritually.

### Effects of the Essential Oils

The sleep-enhancing essential oils save the day. They offer a restful and refreshing night's sleep without all the side effects of medication. These sedating oils trigger a gentle, relaxed state that allows the natural sleep cycle to take over. Most of the plants recommended here calm and deepen the breath, thus relaxing the body. They also are warming. Some of the herbal teas serve as a calming digestive—especially effective when insomnia is caused by a too-large and spicy meal right before bed. Most of the essential oils are especially healing to the skin; we can guess that this plays a part in soothing the body into restfulness.

These selected essential oils guide the body to a natural and restful sleep. They do not interfere with the body's natural rhythms, and some even help induce the dream state. Used in herbal pillows and diffusers, they are gentle. Lavender and chamomile pillows and diffusions may even be used in children's rooms to lull infants. These essential oils are powerful reminders that in the world of plants, we can find solutions to many problems.

## *Setting the Mood for Restful Sleep*

If you are experiencing a troubled night, or anticipate one, you can quickly and easily put yourself into a relaxed and restful state. The essential oils in this chapter work fast, often within 15 to 20 minutes. Be warned that they are the opposite of the aphrodisiacs; they dispel any sexual thoughts for the evening. Make sure that's what you want.

While I have placed lavender in the chapter on depression (chapter 3), I must mention it in this chapter. It is one of the most versatile, gentle, yet effective of the essential oils. It is a powerful relaxant as well as sleep aid (I have used it on many sleepless nights myself). Be sure to think of adding lavender to your blend if you feel mild depression may be a cause of your restless nights. The link between depression and insomnia may be the reason that lavender is especially suited to blending with all the essential oils listed here.

If you experience one night of sleeplessness, try to "set the mood" for perhaps the next 3 days, to see if you can ease your body back into its natural rhythm. After 3 days, abstain in order to check your progress. You should find that your sleep is sound and restful and stays that way for some time. If it does not, put yourself back on therapy. Remember, if the insomnia lasts longer than 3 weeks, you may have a sleep disorder.

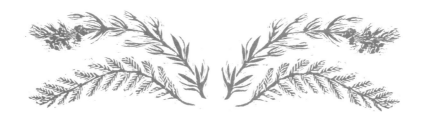

### *Tips for a Good Night's Sleep*

Here are some tips to help the essential oils do their work.

- Make sure activities before bedtime are relaxing. Turn the lights low or use candlelight. Read, listen to soothing music, or enjoy the relaxing benefits of snuggle time with loved ones. Try to avoid bill-paying, arguments, and action-packed movies.

- Don't focus on sleeping. If you can't sleep, try one of the aromatherapy suggestions, and, while you wait for it to take effect, get out of the bedroom. Read, concentrate on a quiet hobby such as hand sewing, or do a jigsaw puzzle. When sleepiness hits, go back to bed.

- Don't overeat just before bedtime, and stay away from alcohol, caffeine, and spicy or fermented foods. It isn't a good idea to go to bed hungry, either; a snack with warm milk or one of the herbal teas listed here will give you a warm, comforting feeling that will help you slow down. Scientific studies have confirmed that carbohydrates, especially refined carbohydrates (just an ounce or two), help you sleep, while protein helps keep you alert and awake.

❦ Try to get into a sleep routine. Go to bed at the same time every night, and get up at the same time every morning.

❦ Learn the technique called progressive relaxation (described by Michael T. Murray, N.D., in *Natural Alternatives to Over-the-Counter & Prescription Drugs*. Tense one muscle for a few seconds, then release it. Do this with each muscle of the body in turn, working your way down from the face and neck all the way to the toes. This is supposed to induce a deeply relaxing state conducive to sleep, especially when the process is repeated several times.

## *Application*

For a full night of restful sleep, choose one of these ways of using the essential oils or herbs.

### Inhalation

#### *Simple Scents*

Inhalation can be especially effective for children and the elderly. One or two drops of the most gentle scents (lavender, chamomile, clary sage, or mandarin orange) on the front collar of pajamas or nightgown will have a calming effect as the scent is inhaled. Plan to do this a half-hour before bedtime. You may also use a room diffuser in the bedroom before bedtime. Once the air is scented, the apparatus can be put away. Remember, you don't want to overwhelm the senses, merely guide them.

#### *Scented Candles*

Add several drops of essential oil to the hot melted wax of a candle as it burns. Keep the volatile oil away from the burning wick. You can do this with several different candles, about 45 minutes before bedtime, as the family watches TV. As the candles burn, the scent will be released into the air, and the whole family will be ready to go to bed.

#### *Sleep Pillows*

In the old days, sleep pillows filled with scented herbs were used to lull the one who lay upon them into blissful oblivion. The kings of England had them stuffed with hops, chamomile, lavender, and dill. You can make your own sleep pillows by constructing little pillow pads to slip between the pillow and the pillowcase. Keep them handy for anyone who needs one.

Take a large handkerchief (edged with lace or ribbon, if you like; plain pillows are best for infants). Fold it in half and stitch around the edges, leaving a 2-inch (5-cm) gap. Turn it right side out and stuff it with a little quilt batting (for softness, not puffiness, as you want it to lie relatively flat). Next, take a handful of dried lavender buds, dried rose petals, or any relaxing herb and put it inside the pillow. Make sure the herbs are fresh and very fragrant. Stitch the opening closed. Now place 2 to 3 drops (1 drop for infants) of an essential oil or blend on the sleep pillow. Slip it between the pillow and case or lay it near the head. The essential oil scent should last several nights. The pillow can then be put away until needed again, when you merely refresh it with another 2 to 3 drops of essential oil. The pillow should last a year before the dried herbs need to be replaced.

## Absorption

### Foot Massage

What could be a more relaxing way to spend the evening than to sit back and let someone give you a luxurious foot rub with a scented massage oil? (If you have no one to do it for you, it is relaxing to give it to yourself.) You inhale the scent at the same time as you absorb it through the skin.

Take 2 teaspoons (10 ml) of a vegetable oil (like olive, sweet almond, or peanut), and add 2 to 4 drops of essential oil (2 for children and the elderly), mixing well. Warm half the oil in your hand, and apply it to one foot. Rub it in, and massage every inch (or centimeter) of the foot from toe to heel, working for at least 5 minutes and letting the oil be absorbed. Wipe off any excess, then do the same for the other foot with the other half of the oil.

### Scented Baths

Take scented baths close to the time you want to go to sleep, as you may feel their effects quickly. The water should not be too hot, just warm. Add 5 to 10 drops of essential oil or a blend. Swish it around well before getting in. Soak no more than 15 to 20 minutes.

## Ingestion

### Herbal Teas

Herbal teas are especially good for warming you inside. They also help you unwind after a demanding day. Several kinds are good for inducing relaxation and overcoming insomnia. Drink no more than 2 cups in an evening.

## Catnip  *(Nepeta cataria)*

A favorite not only with cats, this herb is appreciated as a nightcap, especially in Europe. It induces sleep (its volatile oil *nepetalactone* acts as a sedative) and makes one feel peaceful and happy. It is good for headaches, upset stomachs, and nervousness. It is suitable for sleep pillows and makes an excellent tea for convalescents or children, especially if they are suffering from colds, flu, or other infections that interfere with sleep.

Native to Europe, it is now found wild in the United States. The odor is minty but bitter and pungent. The leaves are grayish.

**Herbal Tea**  Pour 1 cup of boiling water over 1 teaspoon (10 ml) of dried leaves or 3 teaspoons (15 ml) of fresh. Cover, and let steep 3 to 5 minutes. Strain. Add honey to taste. Drink it in moderation. Let children sip ½ cup (120 ml) cooled to room temperature.

## Roman Chamomile  *(Chamaemelum nobile)*

Chamomile tea is familiar to readers of Beatrix Potter's The Tale of Peter Rabbit, in which Peter's mother gives him sips of it to soothe his upset stomach. It continues to be popular, and the tea bags are found in most grocery stores. It is the herb of first choice for children. It is a pain reliever and digestive and is good for nervous stomachs. A cup at bedtime ensures a restful sleep.

**Caution**  Pregnant women should use this in low concentrations.

**Herbal Tea**  Use about 1 cup of water to 1 teaspoon (5 ml) of dried or 3 teaspoons (15 ml) of fresh leaves, or use a tea bag.

## Hops  *(Humulus lupulus)*

At one time hops were much used as a tranquilizer. Merely inhaling the rich, spicy, sweet scent can be enough to bring on sleep. Hops have been used in sleep pillows, because the resinous dust of the female cones (lupulin) is a mild sedative and helps strengthen the nervous system. But be sure to use freshly dried cones, as old dried stuff can have the opposite effect to what you want. Today hops are used extensively in beer-making but are listed in the *British Herbal Pharmacopoeia* as useful for restlessness, headaches, and indigestion. They have a high estrogenic content, so the scent works quite effectively on men (and quickly kills any romantic notions).

**Caution**  This herb can worsen depression. Prolonged use should be avoided since it acts as a narcotic if used in excess.

**Herbal Tea**  Add 1 tablespoon (30 ml) of dried cones to ½ pint (1 cup, or 240 ml) of water, simmer for 2 to 3 minutes, and strain. Add honey and drink it immediately, since it can lose its effect quickly. Children should drink no more than ½ cup of this tea.

*Linden   (Tilia europaea)*

This tall and graceful tree is a favorite in France. Its yellow-white flowers bloom profusely in late spring and produce a volatile oil called *farnesol*. The scent is heavenly and attracts not only bees and insects, but humans, too. The tea made from the dried flowers is highly relaxing, and good for nervous tension, stress, and nausea. Warming and sedating, it helps reduce high blood pressure. Lemon balm and chamomile added to linden in equal amounts make a good tea for overcoming insomnia. It is also good for those suffering from colds, flu, or congestion. Nicholas Culpeper said the flowers were a good nervine. Linden also dispels headaches, especially migraines.

**Herbal Tea**  Make a strong infusion by pouring 1 cup (240 ml) of boiling water over 2 tablespoons (60 ml) of dried flowers. Steep 4 to 6 minutes, strain, and add honey.

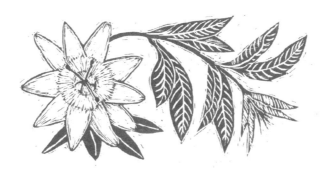

# *Relaxing Essential Oils*

## *Frankincense   (Boswellia carteri)*

**Application**  Incense, inhalation, compress

**Note**  Base, nourishing, resinous

**Background**  Since ancient times, frankincense has been associated with religious worship. It is burned in temples in India and China and in Catholic churches and is one of the gifts said to have been brought to the baby Jesus. Its scent is believed to awaken the higher consciousness. Smoky and warming, it is similar to that of myrrh but lighter and sweeter. The small tree, native to the Red Sea region, grows in hot, dry climates and has compact leaves and flowers. The whole plant is aromatic. It exudes a milky substance that hardens to gumlike beads, and it is this resin that is used. In ancient Egypt it was used as a rejuvenating face mask and in cosmetics and perfumes.

**Use**  Its use in worship probably has to do with the ability of this resin to slow and deepen breathing, something necessary in prayer and meditation. Considered a sedative tonic that elevates the mind and spirit, it helps dispel worries and lets you connect with your inner self. It is relaxing and rejuvenates the nerves. It also is good for dry, mature skin, as it stimulates cell renewal.

**Blend** with citrus oils, sandalwood, and vetiver.

## *Mandarin Orange* (Citrus reticulata)

**Application** Inhalation, massage oils, bath

**Note** Top, fresh, citrus

**Caution** As with all citrus oils, be careful of sun exposure. Wait 12 to 24 hours after application before exposing the skin to sunlight.

**Background** The peel of the mandarin orange is used to make the essential oil (sometimes called tangerine). Native to southern China and the Far East, the mandarin orange (or tangerine) was brought to Europe in 1805 and to the United States in 1845. It has been used extensively for flavoring in drinks, confections, and other sweets, as well as in perfumery, especially in the manufacture of colognes.

**Use** One might call this "mother-and-child oil" because its delicate sweet aroma gently calms children and stressed-out mothers at the same time. It is wonderful for over-excited children and makes adults feel young at heart and joy-filled. A mild sedative, it aids in restlessness, insomnia, and irritability. It also helps soothe muscle cramps and soreness and is very good for the skin. It helps prevent stretch marks. It is a well-loved scent.

**Blend** with any citrus oils, coriander, and sandalwood.

## *Roman Chamomile* (Chamaemelum nobile)

**Application** Sleep pillows, baths, skin preparations; herb in tea

**Note** Middle, flowing, herbaceous

**Caution** If pregnant, use this in low concentrations.

**Background** This feathery green herb is a small creeping perennial with white daisylike flowers larger than those of the German chamomile. The oil is distilled from the fresh flowers, which can be harvested all summer. They must be dried quickly in a cool, shaded place so that the essential oil is not lost. Chamomile has been used medicinally since medieval times.

**Use** Chamomile is gentle and is used traditionally to calm and soothe irritable, crying youngsters. It is put in sleep pillows for the bed or crib. Adults find it soothing, too, and it eases grumpiness, PMS symptoms, mild sadness, and insomnia. A cup of the tea at bedtime, or a few minutes' inhalation of the scent, ensures a restful sleep. Refreshing and relaxing, it is a mild, warming sedative. It has a light, refreshing scent, like apples, and is sometimes called ground apple.

**Blend** with lemon, rose, ylang-ylang, and or lavender.

## *Spanish Sage*    *(Salvia lavandulifolia)*

**Application**  Inhalation; herb in tea

**Note**  Top, fresh, herbaceous

**Caution**  Avoid it if you are pregnant, have high blood pressure, or are epileptic. Use it in moderation for short periods of time.

**Background**  This evergreen shrub is similar to garden sage, but has narrower leaves and a much safer essential oil. Garden sage contains a high percentage of the ketone called *thujone,* which is dangerously toxic, but Spanish sage is quite safe if used moderately. The whole plant has a piney-lavender scent. It is native to the mountains in Spain and also grows in the southwestern areas of France. It is used in soaps and perfumes and as a culinary flavoring. The Chinese like it in tea, and it has been considered a longevity tonic and a memory enhancer for the elderly. In Spain it is regarded as a cure-all.

**Use**  This cheering, soothing scent is good to inhale when you just need a good pick-me-up and relaxant. It relieves headaches, stress symptoms, and exhaustion. It helps raise low blood pressure and clear sluggish skin.

**Blend** with lemon balm, hyssop, and lavender.

## *Vetiver*    *(Andropogon muricatus)*

**Application**  Inhalation, baths, massage

**Note**  Base, nourishing, woody

**Background**  The root of this tall, perennial grass is used in the manufacture of men's toiletries and colognes. It has a deep, woody, delightfully earthy scent that most people either love or hate. Related to lemongrass, vetiver is native to India, where it is grown both to protect the soil against erosion and for its scent. The aromatic rootlets have long been used for fragrance.

**Use**  This relaxing oil is known as "the oil of tranquility" in Sri Lanka and India. It is very thick, so use very little at a time. In massage oils, 1 to 2 drops per fluid ounce (30 ml) will do. It is quite uplifting and deeply calming. Use it for insomnia, mild sadness, tension, or stress. Vetiver makes one feel peaceful when exhausted, it balances and calms the sexual energies, and it regenerates the cells of aging skin.

**Blend** with violet, rose, clary sage, and ylang-ylang.

# Happiness & Joy

*"I have drunken
deep of joy,
and I will taste
no other wine tonight."*

—Percy Bysshe Shelley,
*The Cenci,* 1820

All of us remember moments of sheer bliss. We savor every second when we think back to them. Perhaps we remember glorious moments—a doting father's sweet piano music or story, a perfect wedding day, winning a special honor, realizing we were in love, or snuggling a new puppy. But just how long did these feelings last? An hour, an evening, a day—even a week? Social scientists have surveyed lottery winners and found that the initial elation soon wanes. Other things occupy the mind, and the moment is quickly relegated to memory.

Happiness is meant to be fleeting, for life means change. Perhaps expectations get in the way of our experiencing happiness. Perhaps the negative emotions so fill our minds that there isn't any room to notice the good that comes along. Sometimes it seems that the shadowy, elusive mood of enjoyment will never return, and we long to have the power to conjure it up.

In the last 20 years or so, researchers have turned their attention to investigating the meaning of happiness. In that time, over 20,000 scientific articles have been published related to the subject of happiness and well-being. No one has all the answers, but a few social scientists believe it has to do with being content. A person can be satisfied with contentment. Maybe it isn't an ecstatic kind of happiness, but it is a kind that stays with you day by day. It gives you a balanced outlook so that life's ups and downs don't make you dizzy. And you can live contented while you wait for those moments of ecstasy. It kind of leaves you open.

Have you ever noticed that it is when you are open that little moments of happiness seem to sneak up on you? Perhaps you experience a flood of pleasure when you notice a beautiful sunset. Perhaps you settle in front of a crackling fire with a good book and suddenly just know it is the best moment in the world. A simple smile from a friend, or a neighbor who shares a warm, freshly baked loaf

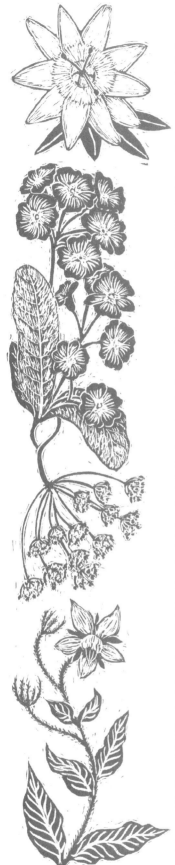

of bread, can suddenly comfort the heart. The greatest moments of joy come unplanned—not at the well-thought-out anniversary party, but as you sit around a campfire.

## *Follow Your Bliss*

But it isn't the sunset or the bread which gives us bliss. It is the fact that suddenly, by chance, we are in the moment. When we live right in the present (a rarity for most of us, most of the time), we aren't dwelling on what we don't have or on past mistakes. We aren't remembering hurts or wondering what might happen to us in the future. We are living totally in that precise moment. It is what the Buddhist monks call "mindfulness." In *Tranquility & Insight,* Sole-Leris calls it "as clear and full awareness as possible of whatever is present now in the area selected for observation."

When you are mindful, cares and woes seemingly disappear. It is when you immerse yourself in the present, whether you are bathing, doing household chores, cooking, or even taking out the trash, that you stand back and become an observer. By practicing mindfulness, perhaps a little every day, you find in time that you are much more content when your mind slows down. You realize that life is merely an endless circle of events, that suffering eventually ends, and that happiness always follows—you don't have to chase it down. Buddha realized this in his famous contemplation under the Bodhi tree. In his *Discourse on the Foundations of Mindfulness,* he taught, "This is the only way, monks . . . for the overcoming of sorrow and lamentations, for the destroying of pain and grief, for reaching the right path . . . namely, the four Foundations of Mindfulness."

As the most elusive of moods, happiness just is. It is a state of being that comes unplanned. But that doesn't mean you can't prepare for happiness, make room for it, and encourage its appearance. At Edison Community College in Fort Myers, Florida, psychologist Michael Fordyce teaches 14 steps to happiness, steps that he has formulated through 25 years of seeing patients and teaching. We have touched on three of them here: lower your expectations and aspirations, get present-oriented, and eliminate negative feelings and problems.

Using these guidelines, you can try to let a little more light into your world. The role of the essential oils is to enhance your ability

111

to feel good. Those oils especially suited to balancing and centering the mind will relax and open you, helping to dislodge negative thoughts. They also have stimulating and energizing qualities. And, because you have to feel good physically to be happy, most of these oils come from herbs which have been used as digestives. Indigestion, a headache, and little nagging aches and pains can take away whatever joy is to be found in the moment. A clean, toxin-free body that perfectly assimilates food enhances your ability to feel happy. So it isn't surprising that many of the essential oils found to heighten pleasant feelings also are cleansing and contain large amounts of vitamin C. Vitamin C is an antioxidant required for adrenal gland functioning, and, like lavender, rose, and sandlewood, it helps boost the immune system.

Besides the six essential oils given here, choose from previous chapters those oils that magnify good feelings and any of the citrus oils. Follow your needs and mood and create a vivacious blend of scents that sends your heart soaring!

## *Setting the Mood for Joy*

The goal, of course, isn't to make yourself happy every day. If you tried that, eventually your body would become accustomed both to the essential oils and to the feelings of well-being, and your response would diminish in both areas. Furthermore, some essential oils are to be used in moderation only. Employ them to highlight particular days. You may add scent to any occasion you wish. Consider a traditional time of enjoyment, the Christmas season. Certain scents remind us of the holiday because they have been traditional at that time for generations. Isn't a Christmas party much more festive when you can smell pine in the air and cinnamon from a steaming mug of apple cider? You could start your own traditions of scent and share them with family and friends. How about welcoming the changing seasons? In spring use floral scents, in summer something herbaceous, in fall something smoky and resinous, and in winter the spicy scents. Or surprise your family and friends any time; cheer up a gloomy, rainy day with something bright and inspiriting.

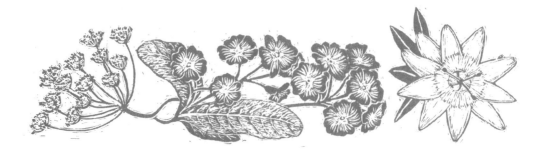

## *Application*

Add bright scents to your day, with one or two of the
following methods, any time you wish to set a mood.

### Inhalation

#### *Room Sprays*

Room sprays are fun to use and an easy way to change the whole mood of your
environment. Use them lavishly. In a good clean spray bottle put 1 pint (2 cups,
or 480 ml) of steam-distilled water, 8 to 12 drops of essential oil, and 6 drops of
castor oil (to fix the blend). Shake well before spraying, and avoid contact with
the furniture.

#### *Sachets*

Sachets, or sweet bags, were most popular in medieval times, when bathing
wasn't a top priority. With their love of anything floral, the Victorians revived
the idea. Sachets are little scented bags that can be put in the linen closet, in lin-
gerie drawers, on the backs of upholstered chairs, in storage chests, even hung
from the car mirror. They can be elaborate and lacy, or simple.

   To make a sachet, sew together three sides of two small squares of fabric, perhaps 2 x 4 inches (5 x 10 cm), leaving one side open. Turn it inside out, and fill
it one-half to three-fourths full of rice powder, potato powder, or cornstarch.
Drop in 6 to 8 drops of essential oil or oils. Sew the sachet closed or tie it tightly with a ribbon. Attach a loop for hanging it up.

### Absorption

#### *Facial Splashes*

Facial splashes are quick ways to refresh and renew yourself. They are especially
nice on hot humid days or when you are fatigued. Choose mild essential oils
that are recommended for the skin, and do a patch test to make sure that they
don't cause irritation. Add 9 drops of oil to 1 cup (240 ml) of water. Store it in a
dark bottle, tightly capped. It will keep about 4 weeks. If you prefer it cold, keep
it in the refrigerator. To use, shake well, pour a small amount into your hands,
and splash it on your face. Be careful not to get it in your eyes.

#### *Temple Rubs*

Temple rubs are good for really trying days or when you feel a headache coming
on. Couples can give them to each other. A temple rub is soothing and relaxing
and also helps the skin. Use cotton headbands to pull hair away from the face.

For each temple rub, take 2 vitamin E capsules and prick them with a needle. Squeeze them out into a small container. (Or use bottled vitamin E.) Add a teaspoon (5 ml) of olive oil and 1 to 2 drops of essential oil. Mix well. Dip your fingertips into the oil, and massage it into the temples and across the forehead. Massage well, and wipe off excess oil.

## Ingestion

### *Herbal Wine Tonics*

By adding herbs to wine, you come up with a dynamic drink as well as a healing brew. Not only are the herbs healing, but studies show that a little wine is good for us, too, and helps to build up the blood. Herbal wines have been enjoyed for centuries. During the Middle Ages, monks in Europe became masters of the art, for they tended both grapes and herb gardens. The tonic elixirs which "made the heart merry" became the basis of their healing repertory.

To concoct your own, use red or white wine, according to your taste. Add orange peel, lemon peel, or spices. It goes without saying that these drinks are reserved for adults, and pregnant women should avoid them. Take a 1-ounce (30-ml) shot glass or a small cordial-glassful, no more than three times a day. This makes a good aperitif or after-dinner cordial. Remember to sip it slowly. If you put an attractive label on a bottle of herbal wine and tie a ribbon or piece of raffia around the neck, it makes an excellent gift of good cheer.

Here are five different herbs to use in wine tonics.

### *Barberry   (Berberis vulgaris)*

Dried barberries taste like lemonade and are very high in vitamin C. In ancient Egypt a syrup of barberries and fennel was made as a tonic against the plague. It improves the appetite, restores the body, is stimulating and renewing, and makes one feel calm and content.

### *Fennel   (Foeniculum vulgare)*

Fennel seed has a strong, sweet, aniselike taste. A great digestive, it soothes the stomach, helps digestion, and eases flatulence. It is a cleansing tonic, a blood purifier, and a mild stimulant. It has been used for centuries as a slimming aid.

**Barberry-Fennel Wine Tonic** Take 1 tablespoon (30 ml) of dried barberries and 1 tablespoon (30 ml) of dried fennel seeds (crushed lightly). Gently warm a fine white wine (be careful, it's flammable) and pour it into a clean Mason jar

114

with a tight lid. Add the herbs and close it tightly. Let it steep for a month, strain it through a coffee filter, and rebottle.

### Licorice Root  (Glycyrrhiza glabra)

This aromatic root has the familiar sweet licorice taste. It makes a good digestive and thirst-quenching tonic. Antiallergenic and antiinflammatory, it is a great detoxicant and a tonic for the whole body. Good for depressive personalities, it has been found to stimulate the adrenal cortex. It boosts energy.

**Caution**  Avoid this if you have high blood pressure or heart problems. It can cause fluid retention if overused.

**Licorice Wine Tonic**  Add a piece of licorice root (mashed lightly) to a wine, and let it soak for 3 to 4 weeks or until the wine is quite fragrant. Strain. Rebottle.

### Ginseng  (Panax ginseng or Panax quinquefolius)

The Chinese consider ginseng a youth-enhancing herb that enlightens the mind, warms, relaxes, and improves energy and vitality. It is said to enhance the immune system and stimulate blood flow. It has been deemed a cure-all, helping the body recover from stress and strain, elevating the blood pressure if too low and reducing it if too high, and balancing both male and female hormones. It can help prevent alcohol intoxication and relieve hangover symptoms. The taste is herby and bitter.

**Caution**  Don't use it for extended periods of time.

### Sweet Woodruff  (Galium odoratum)

Since the 13th century the Germans have loved their May wines, flavored with sweet woodruff. This herb is traditionally chopped and added to punches and cordials. A digestive and relaxant, it is calming, encourages happy thoughts, and aids in reducing insomnia. It has a mild, sweet, yet musky taste and a vanillalike scent when dried.

**Ginseng-Sweet Woodruff Wine Tonic**  Use 1 ounce (28 g) of ginseng root and ½ ounce (14 g) of dried sweet woodruff to 1 quart (1 liter) of wine. Steep this for 2 to 3 months. Strain it through a coffee filter and rebottle.

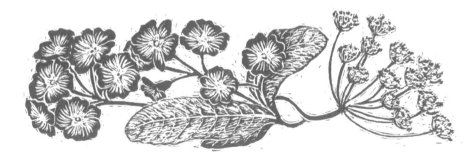

# Joyful Essential Oils

## *Benzoin*  (*Styrax benzoin*)

**Application**  Inhalation, skin preparations

**Note**  Base, nourishing, resinous

**Caution**  Use carefully on sensitive skin. The compound benzoin tincture has been found to cause some irritation, possibly because of the other ingredients in it. The simple benzoin tincture, most often used in aromatherapy, doesn't contain added ingredients.

**Background**  This resin is collected from a large tropical tree, native to Asia, which bears hard-shell fruit. The resin is orange-brown and has a very sweet and spicy scent, almost vanillalike. It has long been used in the East as an external medication for cuts and irritated skin, as well as for incense. A fixative and scent in cosmetics and perfumes, it is also a flavoring. The compound benzoin tincture has proved useful in healing gum inflammations and is a pharmaceutical ingredient.

**Use**  As it increases circulation and is warming, it creates a feeling of comfort. It is mood-uplifting, reducing tension and sadness and imparting a feeling of happiness. It is also good for indigestion, colds, and flu and is healing for rough, cracked skin.

**Blend** with sandalwood, myrrh, rose, and lemon.

## *Cabbage Rose*  (*Rosa centifolia*)

**Application**  Inhalation, room sprays, sachets, skin preparations

**Note**  Base, nourishing, floral

**Caution**  Rose essential oil is very expensive. Because of this, beware of adulteration and make sure you get the true, pure product.

**Background**  Rose is perhaps the most important scent in aromatherapy. It certainly is the best loved, even historically. Persia is believed to be the birthplace of the rose, and the plant is now spread throughout the world. The cabbage rose is used to make what is called French rose oil. *Rosa gallica,* the apothecary's rose, was prescribed for sore throats early in the 19th century.  The symbolism of the rose is particularly complex, and more than 10,000 types of roses have been cultivated. For essential-oil production, roses must be picked at peak time by hand. The scent is sweet and floral, yet rich.

**Use**  Rose essential oil is a narcotic scent that imparts a feeling of bliss, well-being, and deepening harmony. It boosts self-esteem, and some say it enhances inner beauty. Cooling, cleansing, and an energy stimulant, it is com-

forting and sedating at the same time. It is a tonic for the heart and liver and very healing for skin, especially aging skin. So gentle that it is safe for even children's and babies' skin, it is so powerful that only a few drops are effective.
**Blend** with jasmine, orange blossom, and lavender.

## $\mathcal{D}ill$ *(Anethum graveolens)*

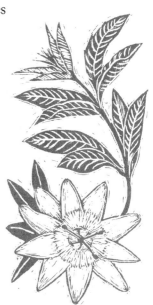

**Application** Inhalation, facial waters; herb or seed in teas, wines
**Note** Middle, flowing, spicy
**Background** Dill, a member of the carrot family, is an annual or biennial with feathery green leaves. To me, it is ever a symbol of summer. It has been used since early times as a culinary flavoring and soothing digestive aid. Native to the Mediterranean regions, where it grows wild in fields, it is cultivated worldwide. The name is said to come from the Old Norse word *dilla,* "to lull." The scent is warm and spicy.
**Use** It is rich and powerful, but more than anything else, dill sharpens the mind, clears the head, and banishes negative thoughts. It brings comfort, contentment, and restfulness. A stimulant, it nevertheless calms the nervous system and relaxes the body. It can be good for stomach upset.
**Blend** with elemi and any of the mints or spicy scents.

## $\mathcal{L}emon$ *(Citrus limon)*

**Application** Inhalation, in diffuser; baths, massage
**Note** Top, fresh, citrus
**Caution** Since lemon can cause sun sensitivity, avoid sunlight or tanning salons for 12 to 24 hours after applying it to the skin.
**Background** The juice and peel of this fruit are very high in vitamin C. The essential oil is extracted from the peel. It is used extensively in cooking for flavoring. In European countries, especially Spain, lemons are regarded as medicinal. The tree is a small evergreen native to Asia and east India and now grown in most temperate areas.
**Use** Lemon is antiseptic, cooling, refreshing, and stimulating. The cleansing tonic is uplifting, and the scent brings happiness and a feeling of blissful sunshine. Also strengthening and good for the immune system, it is useful for a cold or the flu. In skin preparations it helps oily skin and acne.
**Blend** with fennel, juniper, and eucalyptus.

117

# Myrrh *(Commiphora myrrha)*

**Application** Inhalation, skin preparations

**Note** Base, nourishing, resinous

**Caution** Avoid myrrh if you are pregnant.

**Background** One of the three gifts given to the baby Jesus, as told in the Bible story, myrrh was treasured along with gold, the most precious of metals. Folk tradition claims it eases muscle pains. It is a gum resin from a bushy shrub with knotty branches and aromatic leaves that grows in Arabia and Somalia. The gum is collected from the cut stems. It is a common fixative for fragrances in soaps, detergents, and perfumes.

**Use** Myrrh is a circulatory stimulant, a healing immune-system booster, an antiseptic, and an antiinflammatory. It helps balance digestion and regulates appetite. The festive scent of this thick essential oil instills happiness by making one feel open and revitalized. At the same time it is calming and sedating and has a cooling effect on heated emotions.

**Blend** with neroli, lavender, and any spicy scent.

# Nutmeg *(Myristica fragrans)*

**Application** Inhalation for short periods; the spice in potpourris and sachets

**Note** Top, fresh, spicy

**Caution** You must use nutmeg in moderation, and not at all if you are pregnant. Overdosing on the essential oil can be fatal. Nutmeg inhaled for long periods of time can cause nausea, stupor, and hallucinations. Do not use the essential oil in baths. However, the small amounts of the spice itself used for cooking are safe, as is occasional inhalation of the essential oil or use of it in massage oils on specific areas of the body.

**Background** This spice arrived in Europe in 1512 and was widely used as a tonic to induce happiness. Recent research has confirmed its reputation as a good digestive and a treatment for Crohn's disease. The dried seed or nut comes from an evergreen tree whose fragrant flowers resemble lily-of-the-valley. The aromatic nut is usually ground for use as a cooking spice. The essential oil serves as a fixative in soap and candlemaking.

**Use** The Chinese believe nutmeg regulates the body's energy. It is a stimulating tonic—pungent, warming, and antiinflammatory. With a mellow scent, it relieves pain, enhances loving feelings, and encourages sound sleep. Use 10 drops in 2 teaspoons (10 ml) of a carrier oil, like sweet almond, for massage. It will both lift spirits and help reduce muscle pain.

**Blend** with Peru balsam, linden, and mandarin orange

118

# CHAPTER TWELVE

# Releasing Your Creativity

"Blessed is he who has found his work; let him ask no other blessedness."

—Thomas Carlyle, 1795–1881, *Past & Present*

When we think of creativity, we think of people like Kerouac, Picasso, or Einstein. We see them as perhaps eccentrics, but large-souled eccentrics who knew how to take hold of life and squeeze every ounce of living from it. They found meaningful work, work that gave them endless pleasure and rewards.

We've developed a myth about creativity. We think of it as a mystical state bestowed by a divine touch that honors only a few special people. But researchers have concluded that all of us have creative potential; it's already inside us waiting to get out. Why, then, do most of us complain that we aren't creative? Somehow creative people subconsciously know how to reach their artistic and inventive side. Conscious techniques of doing this have been developed, however, and those who can't do so instinctively can learn to tap their creative springs and transform their lives, at least at times, from the ordinary into the extraordinary. Certain essential oils encourage and enhance the flow of creativity. We will suggest ways of using them in conjunction with various methods of opening up the mind.

## Creativity: Myth, Art & Reality

Living a fulfilling life also improves one's health and chances of longevity. Doctors recommend to retirees that they take up hobbies and remain active. The immune system is more likely to function at its best if the body keeps moving and the mind remains stimulated. So many people are mired in the rut of day-to-day events and may not even know how to extract pleasure from life. Living like that leads to boredom, depression, listlessness, and self-pity. To be well balanced, one must exercise all one's abilities, including the creative urge.

119

*Creativity* can be defined as the ability to generate new ideas or find new ways to solve problems. Researchers have drawn a profile of people who are naturally creative. They are self-motivated, love risk, and delight in novelty. They are eager to grab new ideas and do something with them. Many inventors have first visualized a design in a dream and later turned it into a product. Writers scribble notes and scraps of conversation on candy wrappers, napkins, and even table-cloths.

So, first step, keep a journal of feelings, thoughts, and dreams. Second, make room for creative musing by giving yourself time alone. Daydreaming often means entertaining the creative process. Find time to fantasize in daily life. Third, be brave enough to try new things; this will help stretch your imagination. Assume a new hobby or take a class. Fourth, become thick-skinned about criticism and failure. "By perseverence," Charles Spurgeon observed, "the snail reached the Ark." Many an inventor, writer, or artist has built a contraption that "didn't fly" before constructing one that really "took off."

And don't suppose that creativity links you with madness. Many creative personalities and original thinkers live normal lives. The spark of a novel idea comes from a healthy functioning brain, if we but allow it. Certain essential oils stimulate and open the mind to creative thought, when used as recommended. Other essential oils have balancing and normalizing effects. So don't hold back from the rewards of tapping a creative self and finding what journalist H. L. Mencken called "freedom, opportunity, and the incomparable delights of self-expression."

## Setting the Mood for Creativity

Try diffusing essential oils through the air during an artistic process like sculpting, painting, or composing music. Incense has been used for centuries to obtain spiritual insight during meditation and prayer. Some New Age thinkers believe certain scents enhance hypnotic states and help uncover one's psychic talents. But most of us merely want to tap inner resources to solve problems in our lives.

*Brainstorming* is a good way to do this, and it can be successfully combined with use of essential oils. Barbara Sher in *Wishcraft: How to Get What You Really Want* (1979) describes the technique. Sit down and decide that you are going to let all kinds of ideas flow (the good, the bad, and the ugly). Get as silly and crazy a you like, to open up the childlike quality associated with creativity. A really grand answer often comes from combining several of the best ideas, Sher observes.

You can brainstorm alone or in a group. To open the mind, choose an essential oil or blend and begin applying it (diffusion is a good way). Write your problem at the top of a sheet of paper. List your solutions, giving yourself a time limit of, say, 10 to 20 minutes. In a group session, each person makes a list, and at the end of the time limit, all ideas are read aloud. Inexperienced people and children are often terrific at brainstorming, Sher says. "Playing with ideas is the world's best party game." Diffuse heavenly scents through the room as people gather, and be prepared to receive unusual and creative solutions.

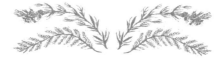

# Application

## Inhalation

### Lightbulbs & Diffusers

A few drops of essential oil on a burning lightbulb, or a scented lightbulb ring (available from an aromatherapy supplier) placed on a lit bulb, will scent a whole room. So will a diffuser, a potpourri burner, or even a few drops of scent in a small pan of water on a hotplate. And don't forget direct inhalation. Place a few drops on a cotton ball. Inhale deeply for a minute or so, go back to work, and inhale again when you feel the need. In a brainstorming session, if you are not scenting the whole room, pass the scented cotton ball around.

## Absorption

When you feel really pressured to perform or come up with new ideas, use an absorption technique, a cool forehead compress, a lukewarm bath, or a neck rub with scented cream.

### Cool Forehead Compress

Set aside a half hour to be by yourself. Fill a basin with ice-cold water and add 2 to 6 drops of an essential oil or a blend. Mix thoroughly; then soak a washcloth in the cool water and wring it out well. Lie down and place the cloth over your forehead. You will be inhaling the scent at the same time that you absorb the oil through your skin into the bloodstream. Every 10 minutes during this half hour, resoak the compress, wring it out, and return it to your forehead.

### Lukewarm Bath

Since the bath should be both relaxing and stimulating, use lukewarm water. To a half-filled tub, add 5 to 10 drops of one or a blend of the essential oils in this chapter that are recommended for the skin. Swish the water around to mix it, and soak yourself for 15 to 20 minutes.

### Neck Rub

A neck rub is very good for those times when you have been hard at work—at the computer, painting, or concentrating steadily on anything—and you need a break to reinspire yourself as well as ease your aching shoulders and neck. To 8 ounces (227 g) of unscented facial cream, add 1 teaspoon (5 ml) of essential oil. Mix very well. Keep this tightly capped, and use it whenever you need it. Rub it gently into the skin of your sore neck and tense shoulders. The essential oil will be absorbed, and the pleasant scent will surround you as you work.

## Ingestion

### Tinctures & Tonics

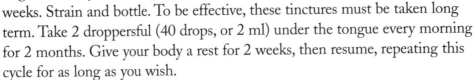

Two herbs, ginkgo and gotu kola, are useful for strengthening the mind and body. They have even been associated with increased life span. Make tinctures from them for a rejuvenating brain tonic.

**Ginkgo & Gotu Kola Tincture** Add ½ ounce (7 g) of dried material to 1 pint (2 cups or 480 ml) of good brandy. Cover tightly and let steep for 2 weeks. Strain and bottle. To be effective, these tinctures must be taken long term. Take 2 droppersful (40 drops, or 2 ml) under the tongue every morning for 2 months. Give your body a rest for 2 weeks, then resume, repeating this cycle for as long as you wish.

### Ginkgo  (Ginkgo biloba)

The ginkgo is an ancient species of healing tree that Chinese monks have cultivated for centuries. The leaf, deemed a brain tonic, enhances memory and regulates the neurotransmitters of the brain so that they increase blood flow and boost the supply of oxygen to the brain. Ginkgo is helpful for learning, memory, alertness, and information processing. It stimulates the immune system and can diminish the effects of alcohol. To make a tincture, collect the leaves as they turn yellow in the fall, or purchase the dried leaves.

### Gotu Kola  (Centella asiatica)

This cooling nervine is an antiinflammatory, blood purifier, and digestive. It is relaxing and is said to restore the nervous system. It aids in reducing neurological and mental disturbances, including learning impairment; aids memory; and helps to balance the brain. Eastern cultures regard it as a longevity tonic as well as an aid to meditation. It is said to be helpful in opening the crown chakra. It also is good for cellular repair of the skin.

**Caution** Do not ingest large quantities all at once. It can have a narcotic effect.

# Creative Essential Oils

## <u>Asafetida</u>   (Ferula assafoetida)

**Application** Inhalation
**Note** Middle, flowing, herbaceous
**Background** This large branching perennial with a fleshy root system is native to Afghanistan. Its strong odor reminds one of a sweet garlic, with a bitter taste. Mostly it has been used as a flavoring for sauces. The oleoresin is obtained by cutting into the above-ground root, from which a juice oozes and then hardens to dark red lumps, which are collected.
**Use** In Chinese medicine it is used as a nerve stimulant. In India it is believed to stimulate the brain and help one work against deadlines. It has been called "food of the gods."
**Blend** with orange, eucalyptus, and sandalwood.

## <u>Borneol</u>   (Dryobalanops aromatica)

**Application** Inhalation, incense
**Note** Base, nourishing, resinous
**Caution** It can be irritating to skin if not well diluted.
**Background** This scent was highly regarded in the ancient Eastern civilizations of Persia, India, and China for its medicinal qualities and for its use in ritual and ceremony. Now it is mostly used for ink, varnish, and artists' supplies. Borneol is a camphor. When exuded beneath the bark and out of cracks in the tree, it soon crystallizes. Its scent is a bit like sassafras and camphor.
**Use** Good for mild headaches, the scent is very stimulating to the adrenal cortex of the brain and serves as an all-around mental tonic. It is best when you are mentally challenged and feel exhausted or are under stress to perform.
**Blend** with frankincense, neroli, and rosewood.

## <u>Cardamon</u>   (Elettaria cardamomum)

**Application** Inhalation, potpourri; seeds in tea
**Note** Middle, flowing, spicy
**Background** This costly spice is rich, spicy, sweet, and gingery. It is used in cooking, especially in curry and Middle Eastern dishes. When it was believed that coffee killed the sex drive, cardamon was blended with it to negate this effect. In Chinese medicine it has been useful for over 3,000 years.

Hippocrates recommended it for a wide range of symptoms, including nervous disorders. The plant is a reedy perennial with blade-shaped leaves and yellowish brown seeds. It is closely related to ginger.

**Use** Cardamon is warming, uplifting, and strengthening to body and mind. It gets the circulation going and ideas flowing. It helps clear the conscious mind and helps reduce mental fatigue. A nerve tonic and stimulant, it is also good for digestion and is considered an erotic scent.

**Blend** with orange, cinnamon, and labdanum.

## *Chervil* *(Anthriscus cerefolium)*

**Application** Inhalation, herb in tea

**Note** Middle, flowing, herbaceous

**Background** This delicately ferny but hardy herb is grown in many gardens of North America, although native to Europe and Asia. It is used to flavor soups, sauces, salads, and breads. Chervil is a distant relative to parsley and sweet cicely and has a strong aromatic scent. The leaves can be used for tea; the seeds are used to make the essential oil.

**Use** Chervil has a warming scent, like myrrh, and its effect is slow and subtle, yet cheering. It helps memory retention and encourages one to see the bright side of things. The leaf tea is a good tonic for the nerves as well as for the digestion.

**Blend** with ginger, coriander, and frankincense.

## *Cypress* *(Cupressus sempervirens)*

**Application** Inhalation, massage

**Note** Middle, flowing, woody

**Caution** Avoid it during pregnancy.

**Background** This arrow-shaped evergreen tree has slender branches and round, grayish brown cones. It is cultivated in France, Spain, and Morocco. The odor of the essential oil is smoky, sweet, and piney. The Chinese have used the seeds from the cones medicinally, and the Tibetans have burned the scent as an incense for temple purification. It is also a symbol of life after death.

**Use** This scent concentrates the mind. It is good for those who tend to be distracted or absentminded. It is relaxing, refreshing, and calming, yet bracing. It stimulates circulation, helps regulate female hormones, and eases tension. It is antiseptic and repels insects. Skin preparations ease muscles aches and cramps.

**Blend** with benzoin, lemon, and bergamot.

124

## *Eucalyptus*   (Eucalyptus radiata)

**Application**  Inhalation, massage, baths
**Note**  Top, fresh, herbaceous
**Caution**  Eucalyptus is fatal if ingested.
**Background**  This tall evergreen tree with the blue-green leaves is a traditional remedy for all respiratory problems as well as a healing agent for the skin. It has a sweet yet woody and camphorlike odor. There are hundreds of varieties, and over 500 different types produce essential oil. This particular variety has the best scent and is the most gentle for the skin. Native to Australia, it is a traditional aboriginal fever remedy. It was introduced to the West in the 19th century.
**Use**  Eucalyptus is cooling and helps deepen the breath. Because of this it is refreshing, clears the mind, stimulates the imagination, and focuses concentration. It freshens the air. A eucalyptus oil massage gives you a restful sleep from which you awaken raring to go. Use 10 drops in hot water for steam inhalation in a bowl, or 10 to 20 drops in 1 fluid ounce (30 ml) of sunflower, peanut, or sweet almond oil for a massage oil.
**Blend** with pine, hyssop, and lemongrass.

## *Galangal*   (Alpinia officinalis)

**Application**  Inhalation, in moderation in baths; dried root decocted in tea
**Note**  Base, nourishing, spicy
**Caution**  This orange-red root comes from a reedy plant native to China. It is used as a spice, especially in curries. In India it is a perfume ingredient. The scent is fresh, spicy, gingery, and camphorlike. It is closely related to ginger.
**Use**  This scent helps keep you going when you need to stay with a project, since it stimulates you to stay awake and also aids concentration. Like ginger it is a good digestive aid.
**Blend** with citrus oils, rosemary, and myrtle.

## *Hyacinth*   (Hyacinthus orientalis)

**Application**  Inhalation
**Note**  Top, fresh, floral
**Caution**  You will not be able to obtain the essential oil. I list it here because it is a very useful scent. And if you grow this spring flower, you may want to experiment with extracting your own scent, although it is difficult.

**Background** Hyacinth is a beloved cultivated spring flower with a green, floral, intensely sweet scent. It is native to Syria and is used in high-class perfumery. It is closely related to garlic, onion, and the wild bluebell.

**Use** The scent is at once hypnotic, sedative, refreshing, and invigorating. It helps clear muddled thinking, improve concentration, and inspire motivation. It also stimulates right-brain thinking.

**Hyacinth Tincture Scent** To make your own scent, pick fragrant flowers and remove the little individual blossoms from the stem. Warm 1 cup (240 ml) of vodka carefully (it's highly flammable). Add enough flowers so they are well covered. Steep 2 hours or long enough for the scent to be released into the vodka; shake often. Strain. Warm the vodka gently again and add more blooms. Keep doing this until you get a strong scent. Store in a dark, tightly covered bottle. Do NOT drink this tincture! Use it as a scent or perfume only.

**Blend** with galbanum, violet, and jasmine.

## $\mathcal{L}$ *i m e*   *(Citrus aurantifolia)*

**Application** Inhalation, in diffusers; skin preparations

**Note** Top, fresh, citrus

**Caution** The expressed peel can cause sun sensitivity, so avoid the sun after using it. If you use the steam-distilled whole fruit, you need not worry.

**Background** The lime tree is cultivated in Florida, Cuba, Mexico, and Italy. Similar to lemon in many ways, lime nevertheless has a distinctive scent. It is used mainly as a flavoring in soft drinks. The juice is used to produce ascorbic acid (vitamin C).

**Use** Lime is a powerful scent that energizes, revitalizes, and helps to get the creative juices flowing. It combats listless tendencies. It is tonic, refreshing, uplifting, and antiseptic.

**Blend** with violet, angelica, and ylang-ylang.

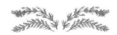

## Metric Equivalents

| | |
|---|---|
| 1 eyedropperful = 20 drops = 1 milliliter = ⅕ teaspoon | 1 quart = 2 pints = 4 cups = 32 fluid ounces = 0.96 liter |
| 1 teaspoon = 5 milliliters = 100 drops | 1 liter = 34 fluid ounces = 4.2 cups = 1.06 quarts |
| 1 tablespoon = 3 teaspoons = 15 milliliters = 300 drops | |
| 1 fluid ounce = 30 milliliters = 2 tablespoons | 1 ounce = 28 grams |
| | 100 grams = 3 ½ ounces |
| 1 cup = ½ pint = 8 fluid ounces = 240 milliliters | 1 pound = 16 ounces = 454 grams |
| | 1 kilogram = 2.2 pounds |

# Index

*My sincerest thanks to everyone who participated in my interviews.
Your time, expertise, and goodwill made this project come together with ease.
—CARLY WALL*